HIDDEN IMPACT

WHAT YOU NEED TO KNOW FOR THE NEXT DISASTER

A PRACTICAL MENTAL HEALTH GUIDE FOR CLINICIANS

EDITED BY

FREDERICK J. STODDARD, JR., MD

CRAIG L. KATZ, MD

JOSEPH P. MERLINO, MD, MPA

CONTRIBUTING AUTHORS

Knight Aldrich, MD
Todd F. Holzman, MD
Erick Hung, MD
Kristina Jones, MD
Edward M. Kantor, MD
Anthony T. Ng, MD
Ann E. Norwood, MD

**Committee on Disasters and Terrorism of the
Group for the Advancement of Psychiatry**

JONES AND BARTLETT PUBLISHERS
Sudbury, Massachusetts
BOSTON   TORONTO   LONDON   SINGAPORE

P9-DBK-063

World Headquarters

Jones and Bartlett Publishers
40 Tall Pine Drive
Sudbury, MA 01776
978-443-5000
info@jbpub.com
www.jbpub.com

Jones and Bartlett Publishers
Canada
6339 Ormindale Way
Mississauga, Ontario L5V 1J2
Canada

Jones and Bartlett
Publishers International
Barb House, Barb Mews
London W6 7PA
United Kingdom

Jones and Bartlett's books and products are available through most bookstores and online booksellers. To contact Jones and Bartlett Publishers directly, call 800-832-0034, fax 978-443-8000, or visit our website www.jbpub.com.

The authors, editor, and publisher have made every effort to provide accurate information. However, they are not responsible for errors, omissions, or for any outcomes related to the use of the contents of this book and take no responsibility for the use of the products and procedures described. Treatments and side effects described in this book may not be applicable to all people; likewise, some people may require a dose or experience a side effect that is not described herein. Drugs and medical devices are discussed that may have limited availability controlled by the Food and Drug Administration (FDA) for use only in a research study or clinical trial. Research, clinical practice, and government regulations often change the accepted standard in this field. When consideration is being given to use of any drug in the clinical setting, the healthcare provider or reader is responsible for determining FDA status of the drug, reading the package insert, and reviewing prescribing information for the most up-to-date recommendations on dose, precautions, and contraindications, and determining the appropriate usage for the product. This is especially important in the case of drugs that are new or seldom used.

Production Credits
Executive Publisher: Christopher Davis
Senior Acquisitions Editor: Alison Hankey
Senior Editorial Assistant: Jessica Acox
Production Assistant: Lisa Lamenzo
Marketing Manager: Barb Bartoszek
V.P., Manufacturing and Inventory Control: Therese Connell
Text Design: Auburn Associates, Inc.
Composition: Auburn Associates, Inc.
Cover Design: Kristin E. Parker
Cover and Title Page Image: © Andrey Shadrin / ShutterStock, Inc.
Printing and Binding: Malloy, Inc.
Cover Printing: Malloy, Inc.

Library of Congress Cataloging-in-Publication Data
Hidden impact : what you need to know for the next disaster : a practical mental health guide for clinicians / edited by Frederick J. Stoddard, Craig L. Katz, Joseph P. Merlino.
    p. ; cm.
  Includes bibliographical references and index.
  ISBN 978-0-7637-6875-1 (pbk. : alk. paper)
  1. Disaster medicine. 2. Physicians—Mental health. I. Stoddard, Frederick J. II. Katz, Craig L. III. Merlino, Joseph P.
[DNLM: 1. Disaster Planning—methods. 2. Emergency Services, Psychiatric—methods. 3. Crisis Intervention—methods. WM 401 H632 2010]
  RA645.5.H53 2010
  363.34'8—dc22
                                                                                              2009012216
6048

Printed in the United States of America
13 12 11 10 09   10 9 8 7 6 5 4 3 2 1

Dedication

*For our families who have helped create space for us to write this,
medical personnel who work to make a difference,
and disaster survivors around the world
who are the measure of our promise.*

Medical Society of the State of New York

Hidden Impact:
What You Need to Know for the Next Disaster:
A Practical Mental Health Guide for Clinicians

This educational guide will direct physicians in preparing and responding effectively to future disasters based on current knowledge from the growing field of disaster mental health. It will therefore reduce the gap in knowledge among physicians about disaster mental health and help them to better introduce mental health interventions into their medical practice during disaster. The information delivered here will bridge the gap between current treatment methods and updated information for dealing with patients in the aftermath of a disaster.

This course will require physicians to take the post-test on pages 243–247 and requests physicians to complete the evaluation form found on pages 248–249 for submission to Medical Society of the State of New York to obtain continuing medical education credits. The final exam and evaluation form can also be found on the website: **www.bcnny.com**.

This is an 8-hour continuing medical education activity and the Medical Society of the State of New York has designated it for a maximum of **8.0 AMA PRA Category 1 Credits™**. It is accredited from May 2009–May 2012.

Learning Objectives

Preparedness

Be able to appreciate how to prepare for and participate effectively in a disaster response within the existing disaster response framework.

Have knowledge of the major agencies and organizations involved in disaster response and public health emergencies.

Assessment

Know the importance of and be able to access the array of screening and assessment tools useful in disaster settings.

Appreciate the spectrum of normal and abnormal behavioral and emotional responses to disasters.

Appreciate the needs of special populations in disaster, including children.

Intervention

Understand the pharmacological and psychological options and limitations in the post-disaster management of behavioral and emotional concerns.

Appreciate the elements of psychological first aid and its application in the disaster setting.

Appreciate the role of collaboration and consultation in the management of disaster-related mental health issues.

Special Issues

Appreciate the legal and ethical dimensions of disaster work. Appreciate the importance of self-care during and after disaster.

Become aware of the processes of resiliency and recovery in communities and individuals.

Contributors

Knight Aldrich, MD
University of Virginia School of
  Medicine
Charlottesville, VA

Todd F. Holzman, MD
Harvard Vanguard Medical
  Associates
Roxbury, MA

Erick Hung, MD
University of California at San
  Francisco
San Francisco, CA

Kristina Jones, MD
Weill Cornell Medical College
New York, NY

Edward M. Kantor, MD
Medical University of South
  Carolina
Charleston, SC

Craig L. Katz, MD
Mount Sinai School of Medicine
New York, NY

Joseph P. Merlino, MD, MPA
State University of New York
  Downstate Medical School
Brooklyn, NY

Anthony T. Ng, MD
Uniformed Services School of
  Medicine
Bethesda, MD

Ann E. Norwood, MD
Center for Biosecurity of
  University of Pittsburgh
  Medical Center
Baltimore, MD

Frederick J. Stoddard, Jr., MD
Harvard Medical School
Boston, MA

Accreditation Statement

The Medical Society of the State of New York is accredited by the Accreditation Council for Continuing Medical Education (ACCME) to provide continuing medical education for physicians. The Medical Society of the State of New York designates this continuing medical education activity for a maximum of **8.0 AMA PRA Category 1 Credits™.** *Physicians should only claim credit commensurate with the extent of their participation in the activity.*

Disclosure Statement

The Medical Society of the State of New York relies upon faculty participants in its CME programs to provide educational information that is objective and free of bias. In this spirit and in accordance with the guidelines of MSSNY and the ACCME, all speakers and planners for continuing medical education activities must disclose any relevant financial relationships with commercial interests whose products, devices, or services may be discussed in the content of a CME activity, that might be perceived as a real or apparent conflict of interest.

The authors and contributors do not have any financial arrangements or affiliations with any commercial entities whose products, research, or services may be discussed in these materials.

Table of Contents

About the Authors

The authors are members of the Committee on Disasters and Terrorism of the Group for the Advancement of Psychiatry (GAP). Dr. Norwood is a consultant to the committee.

Knight Aldrich, MD, is retired from the Departments of Psychiatry and Family Medicine at the University of Virginia School of Medicine, where he had been active in community psychiatry and teaching. Prior to coming to Virginia he had been chair of the Departments of Psychiatry at the Pritzker School of Medicine at the University of Chicago and at the New Jersey College of Medicine at Newark. Dr. Aldrich graduated from Northwestern School of Medicine and trained in psychiatry in the United States Public Health Service. He has been an active member of the Group for the Advancement of Psychiatry for more than 50 years.

Todd F. Holzman, MD, is a child and adult psychiatrist in private practice in Cambridge, Massachusetts, at Harvard Vanguard Medical Associates, where he was also medical psychiatrist in oncology, and at Brigham and Women's Hospital. A member of the faculty of Harvard Medical School, he was chief psychiatrist for disaster services in the Departments of Mental and Public Health for the Commonwealth of Massachusetts and chair of Disaster Mental Health and Disaster Services for the Massachusetts Bay chapter of the American Red Cross. He volunteered for Physicians for Human Rights in Kosovo immediately before the NATO military involvement there to monitor violations of medical neutrality and human rights. He is president of the Massachusetts Psychiatric Society for 2008–2009 and co-chair of its Disaster Readiness Committee. Dr. Holzman volunteered in southern India after the Asian tsunami, working on a rehabilitation program for survivors of torture and human rights violations. With the American Jewish World Service, he volunteered in South Africa,

Ghana, and Kenya on HIV/AIDS education, prevention, and orphan programs. He lectures nationally and internationally. A Distinguished Life Fellow of the American Psychiatric Association (APA), in 2006 Dr. Holzman was awarded the APA's Bruno Lima Award in Disaster Psychiatry.

Erick K. Hung, MD, is a forensic psychiatry fellow in the Psychiatry and the Law Programs at University of California at San Francisco. He is interested in HIV psychiatry and lesbian, gay, bisexual, transsexual (LGBT) mental health. He started an HIV psychiatry consultation clinic at the UCSF Medical Center and in 2007 developed an emergency psychiatry curriculum for the UCSF residency training program. He has been involved in training psychiatrists in suicide and violence risk assessment. Dr. Hung is interested in behavioral problems in the wilderness. In 2003, he joined a medical expedition team through the Himalayan Rescue Association to set up the first medical clinic at the base camp of Mount Everest. He was awarded a Resident Teaching Fellowship in 2002 and has received several awards for his excellence in medical student and resident teaching. He has served on the board of the Wilderness Medical Society, is Councilor-at-Large for the Northern California Psychiatric Society, was a member of the UCSF Chancellor's Committee for LGBT Issues, and is a fellow for the Group for the Advancement of Psychiatry. In the interface of psychiatry and the law, he is interested in forensic issues in the emergency setting, medical malpractice, and occupational issues including workplace discrimination. Dr. Hung has a private practice in downtown San Francisco.

Kristina Jones, MD, is an assistant professor of psychiatry at Weill Cornell Medical College and a voluntary attending at New York Presbyterian Hospital. She is board certified in psychiatry and in psychosomatic medicine, psychiatry for the medically ill. She is a consultant psychiatrist to the World Trade Center Medical Monitoring and Treatment Program at the Fire Department of New York (FDNY) September 11th Mental Health Program at the Bureau of Health Services FDNY headquarters in New York. Dr. Jones maintains a private practice in pharmacology in New York City.

Edward M. Kantor, MD, is currently associate professor of psychiatry and chief of adult services at the Medical University of South Carolina (MUSC) in Charleston. Prior to that he held academic appointments in psychiatry and emergency medicine at the University of Virginia in Charlottesville, where he directed the clinical areas of consult-liaison, emergency, and community psychiatry and served as residency training director. He is board certified in psychiatry and psychosomatic medicine. In 2003, he was appointed to the Governor's Terrorism and Disaster Behavioral Health Advisory Council and is a member of the Mental Health Task Force through the National Office of the Medical Reserve Corps in the Office of the U.S. Surgeon General. Through that group he served as one of the authors of *Psychological First Aid: Medical Reserve Corps Field Operations Guide* (2nd edition, 2008). In addition, Dr. Kantor served as disaster chair for the Psychiatric Society of Virginia and as chief of the UVA-Medical Reserve Corps (MRC). His clinical work, teaching, and planning experience in emergency and disaster services dates back more than 30 years—as a Red Cross instructor, volunteer paramedic, park ranger, and medical officer in the Coast Guard Reserve. In 2006, Dr. Kantor was awarded the Bruno Lima award by the American Psychiatric Association for contributions to disaster mental health education, planning, and response.

Craig L. Katz, MD, is a clinical assistant professor of psychiatry at the Mount Sinai School of Medicine, where he serves as the supervising psychiatrist of the World Trade Center Worker/Volunteer Mental Health Monitoring and Treatment Program after co-founding and directing that program for many years. He also serves as the director of the Fellowship in Global Mental Health at Mount Sinai. Dr. Katz co-founded Disaster Psychiatry Outreach (DPO) in 1998 as a charitable organization devoted to the provision of voluntary psychiatric care to people affected by disasters and has served in various roles in the organization; currently, he serves as its president. His work in disasters has extended as far as El Salvador and Sri Lanka. Dr. Katz received the APA's 2001 Bruno Lima Award in Disaster Psychiatry and has been a fellow of the New York Academy of Medicine since 2007. He is also co-editor with A. Pandya of *Disaster Psychiatry: Intervening When Nightmares Come True* (Analytic Press, 2004), author of "Disaster Psychiatry: A Closer Look," in *Psychiatric Clinics of North America* (Vol. 27, September 2004), and author of several articles.

Joseph P. Merlino, MD, MPA, is a visiting professor of psychiatry at the State University of New York, Downstate Medical School, and is deputy executive director for Network Behavioral Health at Kings County Hospital Center in Brooklyn, New York. He is adjunct professor of psychiatry and behavioral sciences at New York Medical College, where he is also a supervising and training analyst and is a past president of the American Academy of Psychoanalysis and Dynamic Psychiatry, one of the nation's four major psychoanalytic organizations. Dr. Merlino is a distinguished fellow of the American Psychiatric Association, a fellow of the American Academy of Psychoanalysis and Dynamic Psychiatry, and a member of the prestigious Group for the Advancement of Psychiatry and the American College of Psychiatrists. He is chairperson of the Board of Directors of the Opportunity Charter School in Harlem, New York, a public middle school and high school specializing in the education of psychosocially challenged children and adolescents. Dr. Merlino is an expert consultant to the Forensic Panel in New York and is in private practice in Manhattan. He is also author or editor of several books and articles.

Anthony T. Ng, MD, is an assistant professor of psychiatry at the Uniformed Services University of Health Sciences and an assistant clinical professor of psychiatry at George Washington University. He is an independent consultant in emergency psychiatry, disaster mental health, and emergency management issues as director of Mannanin Healthcare, LLC, a US-based healthcare and emergency medical management consulting firm he founded. Dr. Ng worked in the El Salvador earthquakes in 2001, the September 11th terrorist attacks in New York in 2001, the anthrax mental health responses at NBC and ABC networks, the crash of American Airlines Flight 587, Hurricane Katrina in 2005, and the Amish school shooting in 2006. He consulted in the Asian tsunamis disaster in 2004 and the Virginia Tech shooting in 2007. He chaired the New York City chapter of a coalition of Voluntary Organizations Active in Disaster (NYCVOAD) from 2001 to 2003 and has consulted with the U.S. government, the American Red Cross, and the USAID in the Middle East. A member of the APA Committee on Psychiatric Dimensions of Disaster (CPDD), he was its chair from 2003 to 2006 and received a Special Presidential Commendation from the APA for his work in Hurricane Katrina. Dr. Ng is president of the American Association of Emergency Psychiatry and is on the boards of the American Association of Community Psychiatrists and Mental Health America. Dr. Ng is also the current secretary for the Disaster Section of the World Psychiatric Association.

Ann E. Norwood, MD, is senior associate at the Center for Biosecurity of the University of Pittsburgh Medical Center. She is a retired Army colonel, who served as associate chair of psychiatry at the Uniformed Services University of the Health Sciences (USUHS) until she was transferred to join the Office of Public Health Emergency Preparedness (now the Office of the Assistant Secretary for Preparedness and Response) at the Department of Health and Human Services (HHS) as senior advisor for Public Health Risk Communication in 2003. She retired from the Army in 2004 and continued in her position as a civilian until 2007. Dr. Norwood has written and spoken extensively on the psychological, behavioral, and social effects of trauma and violence with a special focus on chemical, biological, radiological, nuclear, and explosive (CBRNE) risks; communication; and military issues. She co-edited *Terrorism and Disaster: Individual and Community Mental Health Interventions* (Cambridge University Press, 2003), *Bioterrorism: Psychological and Public Health Interventions* (Cambridge University Press, 2004), and *Trauma and Disaster: Responses and Management* (Cambridge University Press, 2003), a volume in the American Psychiatric Association's Review of Psychiatry series. She served as chair of the American Psychiatric Association's Committee on Psychiatric Dimensions of Disaster in 2001 and helped it shape the response to the terrorist attacks. She serves on the HHS National Biodefense Science Board's Mental Health Subcommittee.

Frederick J. Stoddard, Jr., MD, is chair of the Committee on Disasters and Terrorism of the Group for the Advancement of Psychiatry, associate clinical professor at Harvard Medical School, psychiatrist at the Massachusetts General Hospital (MGH), chief of psychiatry at the affiliated Shriners Burns Hospital for Children, and senior attending psychiatrist at the MGH Burn Center. Dr. Stoddard is a past president of the Massachusetts Psychiatric Society and a member of the board of the American Psychiatric Association. Inspired by the groundbreaking work of Erich Lindemann and Stanley Cobb in burn and disaster psychiatry, Dr. Stoddard has led psychiatric training for and responses to disasters since the 1990s. He is a child and adult psychiatrist and teaches medical students and residents at Harvard Medical School. His research teams are investigating post-traumatic stress and resilience; bereavement; treatments to relieve pain, stress, and depression; outcomes after burn treatment; and translational studies of the neurobiology of stress. Dr. Stoddard directs the MGH Burn Psychiatry Program, which receives grants from public and private sources and seeks to advance treatments to relieve suffering from PTSD, depression, burns, and other injuries. He is a Distinguished Life Fellow of the APA and in 1999 was awarded the APA's Bruno Lima Award in Disaster Psychiatry.

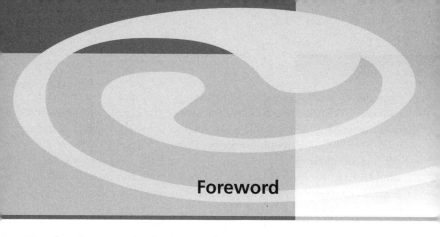

Foreword

We often forget, to the detriment of our patients, that most psychiatric care occurs in primary care settings. After disasters this is even more true because of the number of cases, the availability of services, and the stigma and barriers to care often present in specialty care. The Group for the Advancement of Psychiatry (GAP) has addressed a national need in this publication and is preparing the nation for the future.

Primary care models for psychiatric distress, health risk behaviors, and psychiatric illness are challenging. A number of models for delivery of care are important: The traditional healthcare delivery through consultation, the presence of on-site/clinic mental health care, the use of behavioral healthcare coordinators, and the important role in all these of stepped care are central to primary care where the shortness of time per patient and press of number of patients are critical. Screening tests can help in identifying those most in need. Targeting not only post-traumatic stress disorder but also depression, grief, and increased substance use including tobacco can greatly improve the health of a disaster community and give hope and optimism about the future.

The GAP is leading the way in extending the importance of mental health care in primary care in a practical and usable form. Our nation is better off for their work.

—Robert J. Ursano, MD
Uniformed Services University School of Medicine
Bethesda, MD

In late 1945 while on leave in Tokyo with a few shipmates, I was appalled at the extent of the destruction our bombers had produced. How,

I wondered, could the civilian population possibly have coped with such a disaster? What did the civilian clinicians do to help the survivors with their anxiety and despair? If it was so bad in Tokyo, how much worse it must have been in Hiroshima and Nagasaki.

I had no answers to these questions, and the next one was: How would I have performed in such a disaster? Still no answers, and as I began to contemplate the implications of my ignorance, denial came to my rescue. No need to worry; it couldn't happen to me; I'd soon be back in the States. That comforting thought protected me even through the Cold War, but then 9/11 was something else: It made me aware of the importance of preparing primary care clinicians for the possibility of working in a disaster area, and if it hadn't, Hurricane Katrina surely would have.

The medical library turned up many more accounts of the psychiatric aspects of past disasters than I had known about, as well as a new literature about terrorism, terrorists, and the care and treatment of victims of terrorism. What I couldn't find, however, was what I was looking for: a handbook or survival manual that would help individual primary care clinicians with their personal and professional lives while working in areas of disaster or terrorist attack.

So, I turned to the Group for the Advancement of Psychiatry (GAP). The GAP has had a long history of responding to psychiatry's unmet needs by assembling committees of experts who work together to produce reports that address the subjects at hand—subjects that have ranged from a survival manual for incoming medical students to a technique for dealing with the psychiatric problems of welfare recipients. The GAP seemed the logical organization to produce the kind of handbook for clinician–volunteers after terrorist attacks or other disasters, and, so, after getting encouragement from Dr. Joel Silverman, chair of psychiatry at the Virginia Commonwealth University Medical School, I suggested this project to the GAP's board of directors. I found that the GAP was already considering starting a new committee of expert psychiatrists to look into similar projects, and I joined the experts as a representative of their target audience. Now here is its report.

The report does not provide answers to every disaster-related psychiatric problem. Instead it instills a mind-set of preparation for the unexpected: how to cope when the pharmacy is under water, the laboratory is bombed out, or the computers are out. I believe that this book will reassure primary care clinicians who are committed to service in this area that even without their familiar props their work is doable and personally rewarding as well as socially important. I also believe that it will encourage healthcare professionals who are on the fence about offering their services in disaster areas to volunteer.

—Knight Aldrich, MD
University of Virginia School of Medicine
Charlottesville, VA

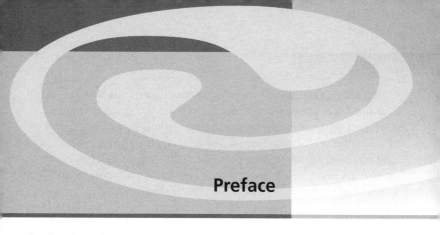

Preface

This book is the product of the authors' collective encounters. We seamlessly pooled our many experiences in providing and teaching about disaster mental health services. The project grew from our concern about how to help medical staff recognize and respond to the often underappreciated psychiatric sequelae of disasters. We are well aware that the absence of an education for, or orientation to, disaster response in our own training reflects the situation at most medical and nursing schools. This is despite the fact that disasters are common and that healthcare personnel are always involved. Additionally, disaster preparedness has been required of hospitals and state and federal health agencies for years, but mental health care has received short shrift until only very recently. As a result, two of us (F. J. S. and K. A.) founded the Committee on Disasters and Terrorism within the Group for the Advancement of Psychiatry (GAP), and we were most fortunate to have our skilled and knowledgeable co-authors join us on the committee and in this project. All of us are academic psychiatrists, and all have collaborated with primary care clinicians and other healthcare personnel in disasters.

Healthcare personnel's entry into the response to a disaster should be neither accidental nor without forethought. Fundamental competency includes appreciating the time course of distress, grief, depression, and post-traumatic stress disorder, and to know the psychiatric and mental health interventions available to prevent or alleviate these conditions. Training physicians about mental health in anticipation of disasters will help them to be more resilient, while promoting the resilience of others, and will help to build community and workplace supports for the ill and disabled, families and children, the elderly, minorities, and other vulnerable groups.

Beyond clinical knowledge, it is essential for physicians and health care providers to appreciate how the systems for disaster response are organized both nationally and internationally. Training and a "badge" of affiliation with an authorized disaster response agency are necessary. And planning ahead for how physicians can communicate publicly in a crisis is necessary to inoculate populations to be more able to withstand stress, lessen isolation, and enhance an overall sense of safety.

We appreciate the thoughtful forewords contributed by Knight Aldrich and Robert Ursano, the helpful reviews of the text by the Publications Board at the Group for the Advancement of Psychiatry, and the assistance in preparing this book by our editors at Jones and Bartlett Publishers.

It is our goal and hope that this book will provide you with useful practical information to prepare you for the next disaster.

—F. J. S., C. L. K., and J. P. M.

What Is a Disaster and How Does It Relate to Mental Health?

Craig L. Katz, MD

In a remote region of Sri Lanka devastated by intermittent civil war and the 2004 tsunami, a priest operates a mental health program for his local community utilizing trained nonprofessionals. With the renewal of hostilities between the community and the central government in 2007, he becomes concerned about the psychological impact of air raids on the children. The priest finds an Israeli study of teenagers and young adults coping with the missile attacks of the Gulf War; it suggests that most of their stress reactions improved with time, with the exception of seventh-grade girls, whose developmental stage may delay their recovery.[1] Based on this, the priest decides that implementing general strategies focused on the situation itself (safety measures, rather than explicit psychological strategies) might be adequate for most of the Sri Lankan children except for some children who may be at highest risk for significant mental health issues.

Whatever the continent or the culture, disaster or other mass casualty events pose a challenge to the mental well-being of stricken communities. Although frequently overlooked, the psychiatric dimensions of disaster rank high among its many facets, as is reflected in some common definitions of disaster. The World Health Organization considers a disaster a "severe disruption, ecological and psychosocial, which greatly exceeds the coping capacity of the affected community."[2] WHO's emphasis on "psychosocial" issues and "coping" signifies an important psychological dimension to the aftermath of disaster. This is underscored by another conceptualization of disaster as *trauma* that overwhelms not just individuals but their communities.[3] Trauma consists of stresses that overwhelm the usual coping mechanisms of people across the age span.

The air raids in Sri Lanka highlight a number of key aspects of how mental health issues and disaster interact and overlap, bringing up points that can just as easily apply to bombings in Israel, a building collapse in a US city, or wherever you may find yourself practicing amid disaster. To begin with, mental health and mental illness are relatively intangible aspects of life, even under normal circumstances. Amid the many tangible effects of disaster, whether in lives lost, people injured, or homes and economies destroyed, it is all too easy to overlook the psychological dimensions of disasters. In this way, a first pivotal step in addressing the mental health needs of survivors is to ask the question, what are the psychological issues relevant to a given catastrophe? That is just what our priest colleague in Sri Lanka has done while others are focused on the more apparent physical toll, in lives and homes, of the government air raids.

The psychological aftermath of disaster can include a range of reactions. Emotional reactions to a catastrophic event are to be expected. Everyone is touched by a disaster in some way. On the other hand, these reactions can become burdensome, whether in the amount of distress they cause or the time they last. Individual symptoms like insomnia pose a problem in the immediate aftermath of disaster, whereas with the passage of time from days to weeks or even months, persistent symptoms become more likely to reflect continuous grief or an underlying disorder, such as an attachment disorder in a child, clinical depression, post-traumatic stress disorder (PTSD), or substance abuse problems.

The example from Sri Lanka also highlights the well-established finding that significant mental health sequelae result not just from exposure to a disaster but from the interaction of that exposure with an individual's vulnerabilities. Thankfully, most people who survive or bear witness to a disaster do not develop conditions like PTSD, and focusing on mental health does not imply that all emotional reactions to a disaster are pathological. However, the chances that someone does develop significant psychiatric sequelae are greatly heightened by well-established risk factors. These include a prior psychiatric history, prior trauma, difficulties in one's life before the disaster, and insufficient social support after the event.[4] Injuries create a particularly heightened risk for an adverse mental health outcome in disaster survivors.

Our Sri Lankan colleague's inquiry was addressed using research from Israel, which raises the issue of the generalizability of the information we have about mental health. The overwhelming majority of mental health research has been conducted in Western and developed countries, including intervention studies.[5] Therefore, a mental health–focused clinician needs to at least consider whether a relatively reassuring finding in Israel—that most of their subjects recovered from their stress reactions with the passage of weeks—translates into information relevant to Sri Lankans. Transcultural issues deserve consideration. Likewise, the Israeli study was conducted with teenagers and young adults, meaning its findings may not apply to younger children at a different development stage with different needs.

When turning our attention from identifying disaster-related mental health needs to addressing them, at least part of the answer to the question posed about the Sri Lankan air raids' psychological toll on children actually lies in the physical realm. Their psychological needs may in part be best addressed by first addressing their general safety. Safety measures as simple as "duck and cover" may save many lives.[6] At the same time, the existence of such measures has a psychological impact. Their implementation reduces lives lost, which itself reduces the strain of war. And communicating and practicing such basic measures helps to convey a sense of security and control for a community, especially for its children who are looking to adults to restore some sense of order to the situation.

The implication of this for clinicians like yourself is that you do not have to implement explicit mental health measures in order to address the mental health of disaster survivors. As will be discussed later in this book, "psychological first aid" encompasses a number of basic interventions whereby early and typically nonpathological emotional responses to a disaster can be addressed through expression of compassion and providing appropriate support.[7] Among the interventions of psychological first aid are attending to not only safety but also to the immediate comfort and healthcare-related needs of survivors.

At the same time, incorporation of mental health into primary care practice is considered by disaster mental health experts to be a crucial means of delivering mental health care after disaster.[8] The likely passage of legislation making primary care clinicians the "medical home" for referrals to specialists makes this even more crucial. Even more than in your everyday practice, people suffering under the weight of their emotions are more likely to seek out you, a family practitioner, or a nurse practitioner, than a mental health professional. Or they may not recognize their own suffering as significant or as deserving clinical attention but present with medically unexplained physical symptoms. Therein an opportunity is presented for you to identify a psychiatric issue for your attention and possible intervention.

The primary care clinician's practice of disaster mental health in the acute aftermath of a disaster affords the opportunity to reduce, but usually not eliminate, the burden that weighs upon survivors. You cannot make the world what it was before the disaster, but you can reduce the psychic pain caused by the upheaval, whether through your own medical skills or in collaboration with a mental health consultant. Additionally, although scientific evidence for this still remains in short supply, the hope is that early interventions to mitigate the psychological impact of disaster will reduce the likelihood that survivors will develop psychiatric disorders over the long term. The mental health challenges posed by disaster evolve from 1) the impact phase, within hours of the event, to 2) the acute phase extending beyond the impact from days to weeks later when the literal and figurative "dust" begins to settle, and to 3) the post-acute phase that may last from weeks to months to years after this dust settles. The practice of disaster mental health can extend beyond the immediate aftermath to deal with those long-term psychosocial changes and psychiatric disorders unfortunately wrought by disaster no matter how great your efforts. The primary focus of what follows is the impact and acute aftermath of disasters, rather than the post-acute, long-term effects.

This book will address a range of topics in disaster mental health that we believe are important for you if you are planning to practice, have already practiced, or, as often is the case, unwittingly find yourself practicing primary health care in the context of a disaster. The book was written by disaster psychiatrists for you as a primary care clinician and is organized into three major sections and three shorter sections. The major sections are Preparation, Assessment, and Intervention, and the three shorter sections are Special Issues, Epilogue, and Resources. The section on **Preparation** addresses becoming involved, risk communication, roughing it, self-care, and the disaster response system. The section on **Assessment** includes chapters on assessment of suicidality, screening for mental health issues, children and families, medically unexplained symptoms, difficult encounters, special populations, and bereavement. The last major section of the book, **Intervention**, aims to provide therapeutic guidance through its chapters on psychological first aid, working with responders, social interventions, psychological interventions, psychopharmacology, collaborative care, staff support, and international perspectives. The section on **Special Issues** includes topics that bridge all of the previous sections, including tele-behavioral health, liability issues, and ethics. In the **Epilogue**, we attempt to bring the experience of a primary clinician to a kind of closure in Life After the Disaster: Follow-Up, Resilience, and Recovery and end with a brief synopsis of the book. The chapter on **Resources** is a goldmine of places to find more material and the latest information relating to the chapters, many of them on web sites.

As mental health uniquely encompasses emotional, behavioral, and cognitive aspects of the human experience, different chapters may discuss "mental health" or "behavioral health" as well as "psychiatric," "psychological," or even "psychosocial" interventions. You will be referred to helpful web sites, downloads, and other resources wherever possible. Case examples will help to exemplify crucial situations and challenges in disaster mental health, and the unfolding experiences of "Peter" the primary care provider are threaded through many of these.

It is not by accident that this book begins with a section on *preparation* for disaster work. Wherever possible, it will be helpful for you, the health professional, to familiarize yourself with the disaster response system in your community, in the all-important spirit of "preparing for the worst but hoping for the best." Such knowledge will help you to be not only more effective but likely more emotionally prepared for working in a disaster setting. The unremitting chaos, horror, and pathos of communities stricken with severe disasters makes it especially important for healthcare responders to prepare psychologically for what may lie ahead.

References

1. Klingman A. Stress reactions of Israeli youth during the Gulf War: A quantitative study. *Professional Psycholog Res Pract.* 1992;23(6):521–527.

2. World Health Organization. *Psychosocial Consequences of Disaster: Prevention and Management.* Geneva: WHO; 1992.

3. Ursano R, McCaughey B, Fullerton C. *Community Responses to Trauma and Disaster.* Cambridge: Cambridge University Press; 1995.

4. Katz CL, Pellegrino L, Pandya A, Ng A, DeLisi L. Research on psychiatric outcomes subsequent to disaster: A review of the literature. *Psychiat Res.* 2002;110(3):201–217.

5. Patel V, Araya R, Chaterjee S, Chrisholm D, Cohen A, De Silva M, et al. Treatment and prevention of mental disorders in low-income and middle-income countries. *Lancet.* 2007; 370:991–1005.

6. Orient J. Expedient civil defense. Available at: **http://www.physiciansforcivil defense.org/sjtrans.php**. Accessed February 7, 2008.

7. National Child Traumatic Stress Network and National Centers for PTSD. *Psychological First-Aid Field Guide.* 2nd ed. July 2006. Available at: **http://www.nctsn.org** and **http://www.ncptsd**. Accessed February 9, 2009.

8. Blumenfield M, Ursano RJ, Eds. *Interventions and Resilience After Mass Trauma.* Cambridge: Cambridge University Press; 2008.

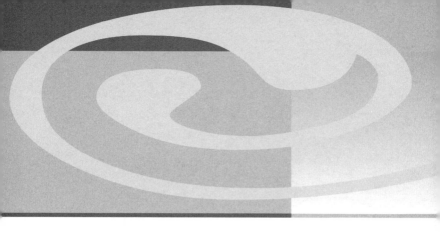

PART

1

Preparation

Section Editor: Joseph P. Merlino, MD, MPA

Getting Involved

Edward M. Kantor, MD

Peter was looking for the right group to join as an internist and thought that DMAT (Disaster Medical Assistance Team) might be the most exciting. When talking to his private practice partners, he realized that it was unrealistic for him to be gone for several weeks at a time in the event of a national disaster. Still he wanted to get involved, so he began to look into the local Medical Reserve Corps (MRC). Peter was assured that the MRC primarily had a local focus and that he would not be expected to respond outside of his local area unless he chose to do so. He also believed that beyond the initially required training, he would be able to regulate his participation as he saw fit.

- There are many local and national opportunities to volunteer. Try to affiliate ahead of time rather than wait until a disaster happens.

- Because there are no absolute disaster medical training standards, joining a group first and following its training guidelines will prevent duplicate training.

- Finding the right way to get involved is uniquely personal and depends on interest, time commitment, willingness to travel, and basic job responsibilities.

Overview

There are many ways to get involved in disaster work. Many volunteers have described their experiences as "life changing" or "transforming." Ideally, volunteer health professionals should have sufficient skills and at least a minimum of training in advance of a disaster event in order to function more effectively in the midst of the expected chaos. Even those clinicians with little experience working in disasters are useful because of their basic medical or specialty skills, the greater demand for services, or the level of need in the event of a complete breakdown in the overall health care system. Most states have ongoing efforts to identify and preregister licensed health and medical personnel.

Lessons learned from the 9/11 events in New York, Pennsylvania, and northern Virginia and the massive response needs following Hurricane Katrina in Louisiana and Mississippi have resulted in many new programs and expanded opportunities for training and affiliation in the United States. These include new positions within existing response groups and even completely new organizations set up to facilitate volunteer screening and participation, such as the Civilian Medical Reserve Corps (**MRC**) and Community Emergency Response Team (**CERT**) programs (see Chapter 2, The Disaster Response System in the United States, for more information).[1]

When you volunteer you should work within your general areas of competence and you should not be required to provide services outside of your clinical or emotional comfort zone. However, predicting what will happen or what is needed in a disaster is not an exact science. As was learned from the events of 9/11, despite mass physical injuries and exposures, it was typically the psychosocial aspects of trauma and loss that turned out to affect the greatest numbers of people. Finding the disaster relief organization to fit your interest, personality, and skill set is important. Duties and expectations vary greatly between different response groups, as does the likelihood of being called out to respond to an event. It is critical to balance your desire to volunteer with the rest of your work and family obligations (see Chapter 3, Self-Care).

When volunteering, it is best not to commit yourself to more than one response group. For example, if you are a volunteer fire fighter or work in a hospital emergency room, you may already have an expected role in your community's disaster response plan, making new volunteer activities difficult or impossible. If you are a critical member of your local response already, you may not want to connect with a national group that is expected to respond across the country or the world.

With these caveats in mind, you are likely to be able to find a host of groups with varying responsibilities that might work for you. The opportunities range from just putting your name on a list to help in the event that something comes up locally, all the way to getting heavily involved in the training, education, and even administration of many organizations. For example, the Red Cross is often looking for Disaster Medical

Directors to support nursing staff in shelter operations and other activities following community events.[2] Also, the MRC uses physicians as clinicians and trainers and some even serve as state-wide or national leaders in program development and response planning. Additionally, federal programs, such as the Disaster Medical Assistance Teams (DMAT), offer the ability to train and travel nationally with a well-equipped and well-trained interdisciplinary team but also require a high level of personal commitment to training and the possibility of more frequent deployment. Since DMAT teams become federal assets, they are typically deployed outside of their local areas.[3]

Roles for Health Care Providers

There are three basic scenarios to consider as a clinician in regard to disaster work. Each has different implications that merit forethought depending on your interests, experience, and current work obligations. These are spontaneous volunteer, locally affiliated volunteer, and affiliated national or international volunteer.

1. *Spontaneous volunteer:* A disaster event occurs and you decide to get involved after the fact. This could be in your own hometown or, as in the case of a major event such as Hurricane Katrina, someplace far from where you live.
2. *Locally affiliated volunteer:* Sign up with a local response group ahead of time in case your local area is affected by a disaster. In most cases this will include pre-registration, some type of criminal background check, and basic training in disaster response issues.
3. *Affiliated national and international volunteer:* Join a national response group ahead of time with the intent of helping in a disaster that occurs someplace other than where you live or work. Most of these groups respond to major disaster events outside of their own region to supplement the local agencies that may need additional resources or specialized disaster skills such as mental health, mobile hospitals, mortuary services, and search and rescue.

Spontaneous Volunteers

People who show up at disaster scenes on their own are known as spontaneous volunteers or SUVs (**spontaneous undocumented or unaffiliated**

volunteers). From early on, even under the best of circumstances, chaos and disorganization flourish in a disaster. With disruption of basic systems, spontaneous volunteers can overwhelm the resources at the scene, adding to the confusion and the frustration of all concerned.

Despite a call for volunteers during or after an event, there are many anecdotes of frustrated physicians and nurses unable to function in their professional capacity because their credentials or individual skills could not be verified. For basic support functions like cleanup, feeding, and other unskilled activities, non-professional SUVs are fairly easy to credential on-site (assuming there is no need for a security clearance). On the other hand, for professionals who require licensing, credentialing, or a security clearance (in terrorist and disaster events), the process is much more complicated and may leave a well-intentioned health professional with nothing to do or underutilized. This scenario can create a major source of frustration for the volunteer and the system.[4]

Because of the nature of disaster situations and the unavoidable chaos that follows, most experts and emergency preparedness agencies encourage advance registration and affiliation for health care volunteers.

Locally Affiliated Volunteers

Affiliated volunteers are individuals who have signed up with a particular group or agency recognized by the disaster response system. It is the responsibility of the organization to credential, screen, and even train the individual ahead of time or through organized, on-scene education known as "just-in-time" training. Due to the diversity of disaster events, even with pre-training there is often benefit from in-the-moment education and briefings on subject matter specific to the event.

Many local, state, and national groups are working at pre-registration systems for medical volunteers, as well as on-scene registration systems for health professionals. Unfortunately, even in our current age of high-speed electronic communication, if the infrastructure is damaged and communication is down, there may not be a way to verify credentials in the moment, and pre-credentialing will be critical to full participation.

Word of mouth from a colleague may be the best way to connect to the local volunteer opportunities in your area. If the right group isn't obvious, try checking the national web sites of the Red Cross or the

MRC. There are clear links to their local affiliates. Most have web sites that explain how to sign up and list the expectations for volunteers. If there is no MRC in your area, there may be opportunities with the local health department or one of the hospitals. With the MRC you can be pre-screened and credentialed without many routine training obligations. The National Guard is often looking for medical professionals, and they take an active role in mass disasters. They are first considered a state asset, but may respond nationally as well. Remember, the National Guard is a part of the United States Armed Services and, as such, they have a significant military mission in addition to one of disaster relief.

Affiliated National and International Volunteers

Here the scene gets a little more confusing. The Red Cross is the most well-known agency for national response, but typically their medical services have been limited. During Hurricane Katrina, the Red Cross and the National MRC developed a quick mechanism for utilizing MRC volunteers to fill Red Cross medical and mental health job functions. This was a first for both groups. Although MRC units are considered local assets, individual volunteers were allowed, with unit permission, to deploy if they had interest. DMAT teams are probably the most highly organized and well equipped of the non-military medical assets. Members of DMAT teams typically train (drill) together and deploy together. During a response, members are considered federal employees as opposed to volunteers. This affords clarity to issues of liability and workers' compensation in the event of an injury.

Recently, the Commissioned Corps of the U.S. Public Health Service has recruited some civilian health professionals as reservists to support disaster and other mission activities. It has not been well advertised, and typically those recruited have been former active duty or reservists from other branches of service. The Coast Guard does not have physicians and nurses per se, but instead U.S. Public Health Service Medical Officers are assigned. There are, however, Coast Guard Physician Assistants in the regular and reserve medical sections.

Some local and state medical and medical professional societies have disaster committees and training opportunities. Instead of responding independently, they are increasingly suggesting that members connect with their local response organizations to ensure that the overall

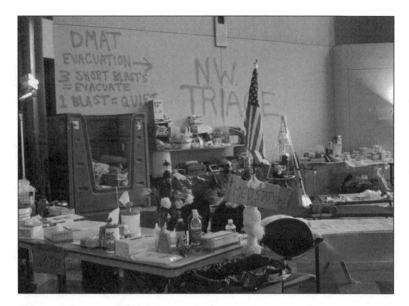

Figure 1.1   A Disaster Medical Assistance Team's medical station after the attacks of 9/11. *Source:* Courtesy of Robert L. Sheridan, MD.

response structure is respected. In major disasters, though, the groups may put out a call for additional volunteers, as happened with Hurricane Katrina, where multiple health professional groups tallied their volunteer lists from their membership lists and passed on willing names to the federal government. If you want to explore international opportunities, take a look at Chapters 22 and 24.

Disaster-Related Training for Health Care Volunteers

General medical training is a complex issue in the disaster response world. Even today, there is no agreed upon standard training across federal agencies, national non-governmental organizations (NGOs), states, or even individual medical disciplines. Many state and federal entities have considered the concept and implementation of guidelines and curricula, but, unfortunately, there is still confusion about whose course one has to take in order to function in a given organizational response.

It makes most sense to first decide what group you want to work with, and then follow their training recommendations. At a bare minimum, even if you are fully qualified as a medical professional, just about every response organization will require some kind of "Introduction to Disaster" and basic "Incident Command" (ICS and NIMS) training. The American Medical Association (AMA) has a series of courses in their Disaster Life Support program. It is not yet the standard; availability varies by region and the courses can be expensive. Furthermore, the behavioral health section is quite limited. Most of the medical specialty professional organizations, including the American Psychiatric Association, offer guides, updates, web sites, and courses on disaster topics. Basic disaster training can certainly be obtained from the American Red Cross. Their courses are widely available and update frequently as disaster response knowledge changes. Their newest course in Disaster Mental Health is up-to-date as of January 2009.

Within the field of disaster behavioral health, there is a movement toward the acceptance of core concepts that is beginning to span both the response agencies and the health care disciplines. Taking a disaster psychiatry or a disaster mental or behavioral health course that emphasizes an "all hazards" approach and utilizes the general principles of psychological first aid can be accomplished through a variety of routes, including the American Red Cross. Some universities, and even several medical schools, are beginning to include basic disaster preparedness and skills training, or a disaster psychiatry course, either as part of their core curriculum or as an extracurricular opportunity for students, residents, and faculty.

Conclusion

Choosing the right path to disaster response participation is a very personal decision. Finding just the right group or the ideal role is something that may require personal research or even practical exploration using contacts found in the appendix. Chat with colleagues and leaders of local response groups to try to find the right match for your personality, interests, and time commitment. It certainly makes sense to be at least basically prepared, whether you find yourself in the middle of a disaster situation in your home area or choose to help out in another community.

Peter has now registered with his local MRC and has completed the basic incident command system training as well as a hands-on class in core disaster medical skills. After attending an MRC general membership meeting, he decided to take the free online PFA (psychological first aid) class through the University of Rochester to improve his understanding of disaster behavioral health. As it turned out, local volunteer process seemed to work out best—at least for now. Until he attended the introductory talk on personal preparedness, Peter had forgotten that someone would need to watch his dogs if he volunteered away from town. As Peter drifted off to sleep that night, with one dog on his leg and the other at his pillow, he wondered, "Who typically takes care of the animals in a disaster?" He decided it was a question for another day.

References

1. Medical Reserve Corps. *About the Medical Reserve Corps.* Available at: http://www.medicalreservecorps.gov/about. Accessed February 16, 2009.

2. American Red Cross. *Giving and Getting Involved: Volunteer.* Available at: http://www.redcross.org/portal/site/en/menuitem.d8aaecf214c576bf971e4cfe43181aa0/?vgnextoid=7bf51a53f1c37110VgnVCM1000003481a10aRCRD&vgnextfmt=default. Accessed February 16, 2009.

3. National Disaster Medical System (NDMS). *Recruitment Information.* Available at: http://www.hhs.gov/aspr/opeo/ndms/join/index.html. Accessed February 16, 2009.

4. Volunteer Management Committee of National Voluntary Organizations Active in Disaster (NVOAD). *Managing Spontaneous Volunteers in Times of Disaster; the Synergy of Good Intention.* Available at: http://www.nvoad.org/NewsInformation/PlanningDocuments/tabid/83/Default.aspx. Accessed February 17, 2009.

The Disaster Response System in the United States

Edward M. Kantor, MD

Peter was moonlighting in the emergency room on weekends to make some extra money. One Saturday night there was a large fire and explosion at a local apartment complex. It was feared that many residents and responders might be hurt from exposure to smoke or fire. The city asked the hospital for a physician to help the emergency medical service care for patients at a triage and treatment center in the parking lot near the complex. Since he was the junior doctor on duty, Peter was chosen to go. On the way to the scene in the ambulance, he heard over the two-way radio that the city had decided to open the Emergency Operations Center. When he got to the staging area near the scene he was signed in and handed a reflective vest that said "Medical Officer" and sent to a roped-off area labeled "Triage." Peter vaguely remembered an orientation lecture at the hospital about the response hierarchy but hadn't really paid attention at the time. Now he wasn't quite sure what his role should be.

- Comprehend the basic terminology used in the emergency and disaster response hierarchy.

- Understand enough about the response system to prevent role confusion and minimize frustration in a disaster situation.

- Realize the importance of the chain of command in large-scale events.

Who's Doing What?

Understanding the basic setup of the disaster response system can be very helpful to health care providers who end up either exposed to a disaster or who choose to volunteer in a clinical capacity. Some aspects of the system are intuitive and can be navigated easily. Others, unfortunately, depend on at least a basic familiarity with the language of disaster response, some common acronyms, and, of course, the basic rules of engagement. Knowing something about how the system works before an event will help to prevent confusion, minimize frustration, and improve your ability to get things done during a disaster. This holds true whether the goal is to protect yourself and your family, support and care for the patients in your own practice, or if you plan to get involved as a volunteer provider in the disaster response itself.

The National Response Structure

The **National Incident Management System** (NIMS) is the federal infrastructure set up to navigate interagency and inter-jurisdictional cooperation during a disaster event. It is designed to be flexible and responsive regardless of the type of disaster—often referred to as **"all hazards" disaster planning and response**.[1] In the wake of Hurricane Katrina, in an effort to minimize the coordination problems between agencies and levels of government, the **National Response Framework** (NRF) was implemented. It retains the core components of NIMS, yet tries to emphasize partnerships and pre-planning, in addition to procedures for communication and control at the time of an event. Under both plans, the scale of an event determines whether it stays local or whether assistance is requested from other regional or even national resources and assets.[2]

Box 2.1 The National Response Framework Resource Center

The **NRF Resource Center** (www.fema.gov/NRF) is an important online reference center that provides stakeholders at all levels of government, the private sector, and non-governmental organizations access to the NRF and supporting documents.

Incident Command System (ICS)

The ICS exists to minimize confusion and facilitate cooperation between responding agencies and individuals. In the last few years, under the federal reorganization after 9/11, the concept of the Incident Command System has extended beyond the emergency and disaster service organizations (EMS, police, fire department, and Red Cross) to include other local governmental and quasi-public agencies such as the U.S. Health Department, public schools, universities, and hospitals. Health care, probably the newest field to join the ICS system, now has incident command training geared toward the need of hospital staff and health care practitioners (referred to as HICS). In fact, in order to continue to receive federal disaster support monies, localities and institutions are required to orient staff to ICS and NIMS and are expected to participate in the local response efforts.[3]

Under ICS, each incident has an **incident commander** who is responsible for the entire event. Typically, the incident commander comes from the agency that first responded or that has primary responsibility for the type of event. For example, during a fire, the incident commander is typically a fire chief. If the fire is the result of a crime or terrorist event, the command may pass to the police or even a federal law enforcement agency. Larger or more complex disaster events, including those involving multiple agencies or jurisdictions, typically initiate a temporary command site known as an **EOC (Emergency Operations Center)** near, yet safely away from, the event. These are typically event or jurisdiction specific and, at least in theory, include the necessary expertise from all of the participating agencies. ICS provides for expanding levels of control, depending on how big or complex the event becomes (see Figure 2.1). By law, certain types of events fall under the jurisdiction of specific agencies. These include airports, military bases, federal facilities, nuclear power plants, and other specialized facilities or special interests.

When an emergency event is likely to tax the regular emergency response system or requires resources beyond the capabilities of the jurisdiction where it occurs, government officials can "**declare a disaster**" and request state and/or federal assistance. Such assistance can include extra manpower and specialized expertise, as well as special funding sources to support the communities affected and to finance at

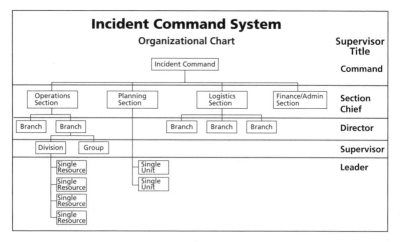

Figure 2.1 Incident Command System basic organization chart (ICS-100 level depicted). *Source:* Federal Emergency Management Agency.

least some of the recovery operations. When resources are needed across state lines, they are requested through a prearranged agreement known as an EMAC (Emergency Management Assistance Compact). Resources assigned through this mechanism often retain both legal authority to function and limited liability protection depending on the activity and the states involved.

Since 9/11 there has been more of an effort to include the mental health needs of those affected by disasters, and more mental health response efforts have been initiated in most states. Caring for the emotional and psychological needs of individuals and communities crosses agencies and jurisdictions much like that of the overall disaster response. It also includes the monitoring and support of response personnel for exhaustion, serious stress reactions, and the appropriate use of drugs and adjunctive psychotherapies. Recent efforts have attempted to integrate sound mental health strategies into the overall response plans and to promote mental wellness and recovery as a component of the core social and medical support efforts. Still, certain agencies and organizations tend to provide the majority of specific mental health care following a disaster.

Major Agencies and Response Groups

Depending on the scope and intensity of the disaster event, plans call for support agencies to either stand by in case they are needed or get involved early in the response. Disasters by nature begin as local events, involving local resources and the local emergency response system. When local authorities determine that the disaster event has overwhelmed their abilities or will become more protracted in time, additional resources are requested by the incident commander through the local Emergency Operations Center. The type of event determines which groups are called to assist based on the resources they bring to the table and their availability in the moment.

FEMA (**Federal Emergency Management Agency**) is the lead federal agency for disaster planning, mitigation, coordination, and recovery, although many agencies, including Health and Human Services, offer various types of technical assistance. Although still working with Homeland Security and FEMA, recently the **National Disaster Medical System** (**NDMS**) and its medical support teams and resources were administratively placed back under Health and Human Services along with other medical resources. These are fully functional mobile medical teams with specialized equipment that can be brought to the disaster site, very much like a military mobile hospital unit. These teams are dispersed across the country. In addition to the general **Disaster Medical Assistance Teams** (**DMATs**), there are those who specialize in mental health and others that support veterinary, mortuary, and pharmacy needs.

Box 2.2   National Disaster Medical System Teams

- Disaster Medical Assistance Team (DMAT)
- Disaster Mortuary Operational Response Team (DMORT)
- Veterinary Medical Assistance Team (VMAT)
- National Nurse Response Team (NNRT)
- National Pharmacy Response Team (NPRT)
- Disaster Portable Morgue Units Team (DPMU)

Source: http://www.hhs.gov/aspr/opeo/ndms/index.html.

The **American Red Cross** (ARC), a national not-for-profit agency, is charged with providing shelters, family assistance centers, social support services, health screening, and basic mental health care during disasters. The ARC is organized by regional and local chapters, each responsible for a particular geographic area, yet coordinated through its national office, enabling it to respond locally to smaller events, such as a house fire, or to larger events, such as hurricanes or other mutual aid requests.[4]

Through the federal **Citizen Corps** program, which utilized several demonstration grants and provided seed money to states and local governments, a variety of locally based, yet federally connected, volunteer programs were begun in the wake of 9/11 and Hurricane Katrina. The two most widespread programs with relevance to the medical community are the Community Emergency Response Team, or **CERT**, program and the Medical Reserve Corps, or **MRC** (recently clarified as the Civilian Medical Reserve Corps to distinguish it from the military reserve programs and the Public Health Service Commissioned Corps). Both began in 2002 and provided funding and program guidance to support the development of local volunteer corps to augment the disaster response capabilities of local communities. Future federal funding for the MRC program is unclear, as the initial demonstration grants have ended. A small stipend program is in place for registered units that comply with basic national program requirements.

CERT is housed within FEMA under the **Department of Homeland Security** while the Medical Reserve Corps operates out of the **Office of the Surgeon General of the U.S. Public Health Service**. Although the local units are registered and connected to the federal government, the programs are administered locally. CERT programs are typically multipurpose and can support the overall disaster recovery with basic first aid, staff support, communication, and other non-specialized activities. The purpose of the Medical Reserve Corps is to register and pre-credential volunteer health professionals to help fill the anticipated need for health care providers during public health emergencies and disasters where health care support is a priority (pandemics, mass casualty, etc.). Although each unit is different, many MRC units have a mental health support component. As of 2008, there were over 729 recognized MRC units with over 153,000 individual volunteers housed in a variety of agencies, including health departments, universities, and even municipal governments.

There is an attempt to create a national advance registration program and single database for volunteer health professionals (known as **ESAR-VHP**, *pronounced EE-SAR-VIP*). Although the effort stalled by 2007, states are still mandated through acceptance of federal support dollars to establish common registration systems that will ultimately work with the federal system. Even now in 2009 in most areas of the country, registration practices and credentialing are not standardized among local groups, state organizations, the federal government, and NGOs such as the Red Cross. Credentialing standards was targeted as a compliance goal for 2008 by the Department of Homeland Security as part of its NIMS compliance program.

As a health care provider, it is best to familiarize yourself with the specific response structure and protocols in your own community, because each locale is somewhat different, even though all basically adhere to the framework of NIMS and the NRF. The disaster medical resources and the expected response can vary greatly by community, and each is heavily influenced by local tradition and the presence of specialized resources like hospitals, National Guard units, or even medical schools.

In the triage tent were several nurses and a paramedic that Peter knew from his ER work. He found out that they had worked in EMS and disaster response for many years. Peter wisely followed their lead in organizing the triage area as well as an ad hoc clinic and staging area to hold those requiring transport to the hospital. At the end of the night Peter sat for a while in his car, exhausted and thankful that his co-workers had been there to help him organize the operation. As he drove home he decided it was time to take the emergency and disaster system more seriously and vowed to retake the ICS training in hopes of better understanding his particular role if needed again in the future.

References

1. U.S. Department of Homeland Security. National Incident Management System. FEMA P- 501 (Catalog number 08336-1). December 2008. Available at: http://www.fema.gov/pdf/emergency/nims/NIMS_core.pdf. Accessed February 17, 2009.

2. National Incident Management System Resource Center. *About the National Incident Management System (NIMS)*. Available at: **http://www.fema.gov/emergency/nims/AboutNIMS.shtm**. Accessed February 17, 2009.

3. U.S. Department of Homeland Security. Incident Command System. ICS 100 Course Materials, FEMA. Available at: **http://training.fema.gov/emiweb/is/is100a.asp**. Accessed February, 17, 2009.

4. American Red Cross. *Preparing and Getting Trained*. Available at: **http://www.redcross.org/portal/site/en/menuitem.d8aaecf214c576bf971e4cfe43181aa0/?vgnextoid=46de1a53f1c37110VgnVCM1000003481a10aRCRD&vgnextfmt=default**. Accessed February 17, 2009.

Self-Care

Joseph P. Merlino, MD, MPA

Peter is an internist in private practice and employed part-time at a local community hospital clinic serving an inner-city population. He lives in a suburban community with his wife of 5 years, Joanna. The couple lives in a single-family home that they own. Peter and Joanna have a 3-year-old son, Josh, and Joanna is 7½ months pregnant with their second child.

Having lived through the media coverage of 9/11, Hurricane Katrina, and other worldwide disasters, Peter's heightened awareness of the need for trained physician volunteers prompted him to sign up with his state's medical reserve corps. As a physician volunteer with the corps, he attended periodic table-top exercises in which a variety of disasters were simulated. On a cool autumn afternoon, Peter's beeper alerted him of a disaster call. Believing it first to be another drill, he calmly called in only to be told he was being deployed to a neighboring state within hours to respond to a massive outbreak of an as-yet undetermined illness. Peter hung up the phone and froze.

- The point of disaster preparedness is to prepare for disasters!

- This includes preparing for your care, the care of your family, and your professional obligations.

- Critical to self-care is an optimal level of disaster training and/or prior experience.

- Disaster training improves resilience and reduces the risk of post-traumatic stress.

Personal Preparedness

Since 9/11, much time has been spent on preparing for disasters. This preparation has included seminars about natural disasters and acts of terrorism, as well as the various steps that need to be taken to provide adequate and competent care to the communities served given the situation at hand. One area not given much attention is *personal* preparedness. That is the topic of this chapter.

Peter's freezing in response to the phone call happened because, despite all of his work on technically preparing himself to volunteer in disasters, he hadn't given much thought until that moment about what would happen to his personal and professional life if he was actually ever needed in a disaster situation. His mind immediately flooded with concerns about who would help Joanna and Josh while he was away. What about his practice and clinic? Who would be there for his patients? With winter around the corner, who would look after the house if he needed to be away for any length of time, especially when Joanna gives birth? It's easy to see why Peter froze after receiving his mobilization call.

The whole point of disaster preparedness is to prepare for disasters! This includes preparing for self-care as well as the care of your family. It also includes making arrangements for your professional obligations. Many volunteer organizations do make information available to assist in such planning, including how to prepare a family emergency plan. You should seek this information out as soon as possible and follow the recommended guidelines that may be specific to your community and setting. Examples of family emergency plans, illustrated in Box 3.1, include making individual cards with instructions and contact information of other family members for each family member to have. The American Red Cross pamphlet "Your Family Disaster Plan" is an excellent tool to help you prepare. It is available at: **http://www.redcross.org/services/disaster/beprepared/fdpall.pdf.**

While making preparations for being called to respond is critical, this step needs to be followed by making preparations to take care of yourself once at the disaster site. This is self-care for responders. In addition to the steps outlined in Box 3.1, Peter needs to familiarize himself with the following self-care tips (see Table 3.1). For more information on

Box 3.1 Four Steps to Safety

The Four Steps to Safety highlighted in this Red Cross pamphlet are:

1. Find out what could happen to you. These are selected questions for you to ask your local emergency management chapter.
2. Create a disaster plan. This describes a family meeting and the kind of information sharing that should occur to be prepared for a disaster.
3. Complete a checklist. This is a short important listing of items to help you be prepared.
4. Practice and maintain your plan. The Red Cross pamphlet provides a simple program to keep you prepared after you go through the steps above.

Source: American Red Cross

managing and preventing stress, see "Tips for Managing and Preventing Stress" at the Substance Abuse and Mental Health Services Administration's (SAMHSA) web site at: **http://mentalhealth.samhsa.gov/publications/allpubs/KEN-01-0098/**.

An important consideration in self-care is how you manage your need for intimacy. Loneliness and isolation from family and friends can take its toll. Keeping a journal, writing letters (if you can mail them), and email (if the infrastructure supports this) are important ways to "keep in touch."

Training and Experience

Critical to self-care is an optimal level of disaster training and/or prior experience. Educated and trained individuals perform better in the field, experience lower levels of stress, are likely to be more resilient, and are likely to grow psychologically in response to the stress of disaster experience.[1-3] Disaster training also helps prepare the responder to deal with anticipatory stress, typically experienced prior to actually responding to the disaster, as occurs in those awaiting assignment in the field.[4] The importance of such training has been well documented in studies that have shown that the least prepared individuals responding in disasters

Table 3.1 Managing and Preventing Stress

1. Normal reactions to a disaster event:

 a. No one is untouched by a mass casualty event.
 b. Sadness, grief, and anger are normal reactions to an abnormal event.
 c. You may not want to leave the scene until the work is finished.
 d. You will try to override stress and fatigue with commitment.
 e. You may deny the need to rest and take time to recover.

2. Signs that you may need stress management assistance:

 a. Difficulty communicating thoughts or remembering instructions
 b. Difficulty concentrating or making decisions
 c. Becoming uncharacteristically argumentative
 d. Limited attention span
 e. Unnecessary risk taking
 f. Becoming easily frustrated
 g. Increased use of drugs and/or alcohol

3. Ways to help manage your stress:

 a. Limit work hours to no more than 12 hours per day.
 b. Make work rotations from high stress to lower stress functions.
 c. Make work rotations from the scene to routine assignments.
 d. Drink plenty of water and eat healthy snacks.
 e. Take frequent, brief breaks from the scene.
 f. Talk about your emotions.
 g. Stay in touch with family and friends.

Source: SAMHSA

are the ones more likely to later develop PTSD.[5] Decreasing anticipatory stress is important in lessening fatigue, enhancing overall performance, and decreasing risk for psychological adverse effects such as PTSD in responders.[6]

Health care providers are trained to identify signs and symptoms in their patients. It is equally important to be alert to your own emotional and bodily reactions. An "uneasy feeling" in the pit of our stomach when dealing with a certain patient, for instance, can be an important piece of data alerting you to something about that patient. Such knowledge is typically acquired through professional training and experience but also importantly from the day-to-day real-life events you experience by inter-acting with people in your private life. Such clues are especially important in the disaster setting where both you and the patient are victimized by the disaster you are experiencing. This fact stresses your defenses and challenges your professional training. Nevertheless, identifying such reactions allows you to take better care of yourself as well as those you are working with.

The psychoanalytic concept of countertransference is useful in understanding the clinician's conscious and unconscious feelings and examining how these facilitate or hinder the therapeutic work.[7] The polar opposites of over-identification and avoidance are frequently cited examples in which the responder gets overly involved (or overly identified) with the victim. They believe that "it could have been me" or the responder avoids the pain of the experience by not getting involved at all. The sources of these reactions are many and include the very "real" reaction to the current situation, the responder's past experiences and emotional conflicts dealing with crises, existential despair as well as a sense of kinship with the victim who may share personal (e.g., the age of your child or your age, education, etc.) cultural, ethnic, or religious identities.

Compassion fatigue or burnout can result when responders do not take care of their personal needs, including adequate rest, sleep, and nutrition as well as breaks from exposure to the disaster site or to those directly impacted by the disaster. Such behavior typically occurs in those displaying counter-phobic behavior—a defensive maneuver in which one deals with a fearful situation by totally immersing oneself in it. Similarly, overexposure to media coverage of the disaster can have the same effect as overworking in the field and should be monitored and limited to obtaining important updates. The endless television replays in which the hijacked jets crashed into the World Trade Center along with the horrific collapse of the Twin Towers left many feeling they were witnessing the death of their loved ones "over and over again." The 24-hour live news coverage provided by CNN and other networks offers sensationalistic coverage of disasters around the clock. Although the dissemination of real-time news is invaluable, the endless replay of tragedy and devastation should be avoided as part of your care plan. It's all right to turn the television off.

From my own work experience during 9/11, as well as working with caregivers during the early years of the AIDS epidemic, it became clear to me that providers shunned sharing information and details about their work with family and loved ones. At the same time, many wished their spouses had been knowledgeable about the nature of their work.[8] Such information can be conveyed to families of disaster responders to allay their fears while providing an opportunity for them to be able to communicate with their spouses and offer support and compassion.

Benefits of Volunteering

Remember that volunteering in a disaster has many benefits. Much work has been done on the positive effects of selfless giving. Stephen Post and Jill Neimark found that people who are generous with their time and talents live longer, healthier, and happier lives. These authors summarize results of scientific studies demonstrating that such giving contributes to mental and physical health by providing opportunities for celebration, generativity (i.e., passing knowledge and wisdom on to others, especially future generations), forgiveness, courage, humor, respect, compassion, loyalty, listening, and creativity.[9]

The National Mental Health Information Center web site notes,

> *Despite the inevitable stresses and challenges associated with community crisis response, workers experience personal gratification by using their skills and training to assist fellow humans in need. Active engagement in the disaster response and "doing" for others can be an antidote for feelings of vulnerability, powerlessness, and outrage commonly experienced by non-impacted community members. Witnessing the courage and resilience of the human spirit and the power of human kindness can have profound and lasting effects.*[10]

Personalizing Your Self-Care

Many suggestions have been offered in this chapter for ways to take care of yourself when you are helping others during a disaster. Of course all of the recommendations discussed here can't always be followed. You may not be able to take a bath to relax while listening to classical music during a disaster, but you get the idea! Improvisation and flexibility are essential in coping with disasters. Use the general concepts outlined in the previous sections to design your unique plan. It doesn't have to be perfect, but get one started and revise it regularly as you think through different aspects of your self-care plan.

Peter will have to get family or friends lined up to help his wife and family. Likewise, a colleague will be needed to cover his practice and he will need to be released, and covered, from his clinic duties. His self-care exercises will need to be regularly practiced to keep him sound in mind and body and able to respond to the disaster at hand while taking care of others and himself. One option open to Peter is to decline serving at this particular time if his assessment concludes that the risk-benefit burden to his personal life and that of his family just doesn't realistically permit his safe deployment. Although this decision would be difficult and would probably raise emotional issues, such as feelings of guilt and shame, Peter should be supported in this decision if it has to be made. What would you have decided to do if you were Peter?

References

1. Ursano RJ, McCarroll JE, Fullerton CS. Traumatic death in terrorism and disaster. In: Ursano RJ, Fullerton CS, Norwood AE, Eds. *Terrorism and Disaster: Individual and Community Mental Health Interventions.* Cambridge: Cambridge University Press; 2003:310.

2. American Medical Association Center for Public Health Preparedness and Disaster Response. *Management of Public Health Emergencies: A Resource Guide for Physicians and Other Community Responders.* Available at: http://www.ama-assn.org/ama/no-index/physician-resources/18200_print.html. Accessed March 12, 2009.

3. Charney DS. Psychobiological mechanisms of resilience and vulnerability: implications for successful adaptation to extreme stress. *Am J Psychiatry.* 2004;161(2):195–216.

4. Watson PJ, Ritchie EC, Demer J, Bartone P, Pfefferbaum BJ. Improving resilience trajectories following mass violence and disasters. In: Ritchie EC, Watson PJ, Friedman MJ, Eds. *Interventions Following Mass Violence and Disasters: Strategies for Mental Health Practice.* New York: The Guilford Press; 2006:37–53.

5. Perrin MA, DiGrande L, Wheeler K, Thorpe L, Farfel M, Brackbill R. PTSD prevalence and associated risk factors among world trade center disaster rescue and recovery workers. *Am J Psychiatry.* 2007;164:1385–1394.

6. Ursano RJ, McCarroll JE, Fullerton CS. Traumatic death in terrorism and disaster. In: Ursano RJ, Fullerton CS, Norwood AE, Eds. *Terrorism and*

Disaster: Individual and Community Mental Health Interventions. Cambridge: Cambridge University Press; 2003:311.

7. Lindy JD, Lindy DC. Countertransference and disaster psychiatry: from Buffalo Creek to 9/11. In: Katz CL, Pandya A, Eds. *Disaster Psychiatry: A Closer Look.* Philadelphia: WB Saunders Publishers; 2004:517–587.

8. Ursano RJ, McCarroll JE, Fullerton CS. Traumatic death in terrorism and disaster. In: Ursano RJ, Fullerton CS, Norwood AE, Eds. *Terrorism and Disaster: Individual and Community Mental Health Interventions.* Cambridge: Cambridge University Press; 2003:328.

9. Post S, Neimark J. *Why Good Things Happen to Good People.* New York: Broadway Books; 2008.

10. U.S. Department of Health and Human Services. *Mental Health Response to Mass Violence and Terrorism: A Training Manual.* DHHS Pub. No. SMA 3959. Available at: **http://mentalhealth.samhsa.gov/publications/allpubs/ SMA-3959/chapter5.asp**. Accessed February 18, 2009.

Roughing It: Preparing to Help in a Disaster

Erick Hung, MD

In preparing to help in a hurricane disaster, Peter asks a medical colleague, "What important items do I need to bring? What if the conditions are unstable? How will I make sure that I plan appropriately?" The colleague tells him to focus on the survivors' needs and not his own. Thankfully, Peter's wife suggests he speak with the volunteer coordinator of the agency, and he emails Peter a long pre-travel "to-do" list for all of their volunteers.

Planning Ahead

Preparation and planning are essential in providing assistance during a disaster. Before you help others in a disaster, it is crucial for you to prepare adequately. Oftentimes you may be traveling to areas of unfamiliarity, either nationally or abroad. Other times you may be assisting in your own neighborhood or city. Additionally, local infrastructure at the disaster site may be limited, unreliable, or even destroyed. Power, water, communications, roads, and accommodations may all be affected to varying degrees depending on the disaster. In some disasters, the threat to local infrastructure may be ongoing or continually evolving.

- Give yourself time to prepare adequately before helping in a disaster.

- Know the conditions of the disaster site at which you are assisting and remember that conditions may change on a day-by-day basis.

- Use checklists to remember to bring crucial items.

In preparing to assist at a disaster site, you not only need to plan for the standard travel to that particular area, but you need to be mindful of the potential dysfunction in that area given the impact of the disaster. Both standard travel tips as well as tips for surviving in suboptimal conditions are crucial. Whether assisting in your own local area or traveling abroad, disaster conditions may require a "roughing it" of sorts as you provide assistance. The following tips are important to consider as you prepare to help in a disaster.

Tip 1: Check It Off Before Take-Off

Before you leave to help in a disaster, particularly with short notice, it is easy to get overwhelmed. It is essential that you plan ahead. The best thing that you can do in this situation is create a checklist. Before you create the list you should factor in a couple of questions, such as:[1,2]

- Where are you going?
- Who are you going with?
- For how long are you going? Could the time that you stay at the disaster site change?
- What is the current infrastructure at the disaster site?
- What is the extended weather forecast in that area of the country or world?

Once all of these questions are factored in, then you can create your list. If you are having trouble writing the list, you can check the Internet to find sample packing list travel tips from people who have visited specific countries or areas of the United States. At the end of this chapter, we have included a standard checklist that incorporates both international travel and working in areas with limited infrastructure. This checklist is meant to be a launching point as you make preparations for travel. You will need to tailor your own personal checklist to the area to which you are traveling and the specifics of the particular disaster.

Tip 2: Documents to Take With You

Make sure that you have all of these essential documents before you travel:

- ☐ Passport with required visas (passport should be valid for at least 6 months from start of trip)
- ☐ Visas for entry into countries to be visited, including those through which you will transit
- ☐ Health book (record of immunizations)
- ☐ Airline tickets (many countries require round-trip ticket for entry)
- ☐ Driver's license
- ☐ Fax, telex, or letter stating that your visa will be available upon arrival for countries that do not issue visas outside their country (e.g., UAE, Oman)
- ☐ Traveler's checks (exchange for local currency as needed at a bank)
- ☐ Major international credit cards (e.g., American Express, Diners, and VISA/MasterCard)
- ☐ Airline frequent travel cards
- ☐ Telephone numbers at destinations and addresses in countries to be visited (may be needed for landing cards)
- ☐ Two copies of your passport and visas
- ☐ Malpractice information
- ☐ Medical licensure information
- ☐ Health insurance information

Tip 3: Sleep-to-Go

Walking into a disaster site for health care volunteers is not like walking into a four-star hotel. Though there may be beds, those beds might not be pest-free. So, it might be best to bring your own bed—a sleeping bag. True, sleeping bags can be cumbersome to pack. However, you can buy a sleep sack, which is basically three sheets sewn together. You would sleep in it much like you would a sleeping bag. The difference is that sleep sacks are made from lighter material that won't take up a lot of room in your bags.

Tip 4: Disposable Is Doable

Depending on where you are going all the comforts of home might not be available—particularly running water. If you are traveling to a third world nation, water is a luxury and not something that every place has. To be prepared, you should "pack disposable." Try not to pack too many things that depend on water, like razors or contacts. Get their disposable counterparts. If you do need to use water to rinse out something (like a toothbrush), use bottled water. Even if the place has running water there is no telling if it is pure enough to drink (see Tip 9).

Tip 5: Pack Your Pills

If you are taking prescription medicine, you probably will not forget to add it to your international travel checklist. However, you should also pack any over-the-counter medications you take or may need. Local pharmacies may not be available at a disaster site. Think about analgesics, antidiarrheals, antimalarials, and antibiotics in consultation with a specialist in travel medicine.

Tip 6: Pack Your Own Power

The disaster site may have limited power capabilities. Make sure that you bring your own power for your portable gadgets like cellular phones, PDAs, and personal hygiene. The best thing to do is to throw an extra pack of batteries in the bag. This way if the batteries fade you have backup power. If you have electronic devices that require you to plug into a power source, think about purchasing a battery-powered power source for your electronic gadgets in the event that power is limited at the disaster site.

Tip 7: Adapt With an Adaptor

When packing for an international trip it's important to pack smart. Take only what you need. The lighter the packing, the more room you will have to bring stuff back. So, if you are looking to bring any electrical items like a curling iron, hairdryer, or an electric razor, make sure it is portable. Also, keep in mind that electrical outlets are not the same throughout the world. So, chances are your cell phone will not plug into where you are going. To help, you should probably pick up a variety of international electrical outlet adapters. Do a search engine search to find out the electrical standard at your travel destination and which local stores carry them.

Tip 8: CDC Travel Recommendations for Health

The official U.S. government health recommendations for traveling are provided by the U.S. Centers for Disease Control and Prevention (CDC) at: **www.cdc.gov/travel**.

Tip 9: Beware of the Water

Diarrhea is an unpleasant ailment to discuss and even more unpleasant to have. It is actually the most common illness people get overseas and is usually caused by eating vegetables or fruit that have not been cleaned properly. Another major cause is dehydration. Fortunately, both of these problems can be avoided if you drink and use either bottled or purified water. If you are unsure about the contamination of your water supply, consider using a decontaminant agent (e.g., iodine) or a water filtration system. If these methods fail, be sure to bring antidiarrhea medications. Remember ice is also water, so if you do order a soda in a restaurant, it is best to order it without ice.

Tip 10: Department of State Travel Advisories

Travel warnings are issued when the State Department recommends that Americans avoid certain countries. The State Department issues Consular Information Sheets for every country in the world with information on such matters as the health conditions, crime, unusual currency or entry requirements, any areas of instability, and the location of the nearest U.S. embassy or consulate in the subject country.

If you are traveling internationally, be sure check out of these sites before travel: **http://travel.state.gov/travel/warnings_current.html**, **www.state.gov/s/cpr/rls/dpl**.

International Travel Checklist

Here are some key items that you should have or consider for an international trip.[3] This list addresses the practical and essential items.

To-Do List Before You Go

- ☐ Get country information
- ☐ Check current advisories
- ☐ Get or renew passport
- ☐ Get immunizations
- ☐ Check health insurance
- ☐ Check travel insurance
- ☐ Check evacuation insurance
- ☐ Check auto insurance
- ☐ Get transportation tickets
- ☐ Make lodging reservations
- ☐ Confirm reservations
- ☐ Weigh and measure luggage
- ☐ Empty wallet extras

Basics

- ☐ Passport and visas
- ☐ Two passport photos
- ☐ Vaccination certificate
- ☐ International driver's license
- ☐ Your driver's license
- ☐ Your medical license information
- ☐ Photo ID (in addition to passport photos)
- ☐ Copy of documentation
- ☐ Credit card
- ☐ ATM card
- ☐ Traveler's checks
- ☐ Wallet/neck pouch
- ☐ Luggage locks
- ☐ Luggage ID tags
- ☐ Travel watch/alarm clock
- ☐ Tickets
- ☐ Cell phone/pager
- ☐ International calling card
- ☐ Phone access codes
- ☐ First-aid kit
- ☐ Pocket knife (to go in checked bag)

- ☐ Sewing kit/safety pins
- ☐ Water bottle
- ☐ Water purification/iodine tablets

Personal Items

- ☐ Dental floss
- ☐ Small bandages
- ☐ Moleskin
- ☐ Medicines
- ☐ Prescriptions (in original containers)
- ☐ Eyewear prescription
- ☐ Earplugs
- ☐ Insect repellent
- ☐ Sunscreen
- ☐ Feminine hygiene products

Miscellaneous

- ☐ Electrical adapters
- ☐ Resealable plastic bags
- ☐ Small flashlight
- ☐ Extra batteries/bulbs

Think About These

- ☐ Address book/PDA
- ☐ Wilderness medicine or first-aid handbook
- ☐ Paperback books
- ☐ Camera
- ☐ Maps of local area
- ☐ Language phrase book
- ☐ Brimmed hat
- ☐ Lip salve
- ☐ Water shoes
- ☐ Bandanna/scarf
- ☐ Duct tape (fixes everything!)
- ☐ Support socks/exerciser
- ☐ Snacks
- ☐ Sunburn relief

☐ Anti-itch gel
☐ Travel pillow
☐ Sunglasses

Roughing It Checklist

Here are some key items that you should have or consider in the event that the infrastructure at the disaster site is severely compromised.

The 10+ Essentials

☐ Extra clothing layers
☐ Drinking water
☐ Food
☐ First-aid kit
☐ Pocket knife
☐ Matches (in waterproof container)
☐ Map of areas (in waterproof case)
☐ Compass
☐ Headlamp or flashlight (with extra batteries/bulbs)
☐ Sunglasses (with retaining strap)
☐ Sunscreen

Clothing

☐ Quick-drying pants/shorts
☐ Short-sleeved shirts
☐ Long-sleeved shirts
☐ Warm pants (fleece or wool)
☐ Fleece or wool vest
☐ Fleece jacket or wool sweater
☐ Wicking long underwear (top/bottoms)
☐ Regular underwear

Outerwear

☐ Rainwear (top/bottoms)
☐ Wide-brimmed rain/sun hat
☐ Warm hat (fleece or wool)

- ☐ Fleece or wool gloves/mittens
- ☐ Waterproof gloves/overmitts
- ☐ Bandanna

Footwear

- ☐ Hiking socks
- ☐ Wicking liner socks
- ☐ Comfortable shoes that prevent blisters and match the terrain
- ☐ Extra laces

Camping Gear

- ☐ Backpack
- ☐ Day pack
- ☐ Pack cover
- ☐ Tent, tarp, or bivvy sack
- ☐ Rainfly
- ☐ Tent stakes
- ☐ Tarp for underneath tent
- ☐ Sleeping bag (in waterproof sack)
- ☐ Compression sack
- ☐ Sleeping pad
- ☐ Sit pad or sleeping pad chair kit
- ☐ Stove and fuel
- ☐ Matches/lighter
- ☐ Cook set, dishes
- ☐ Cooking/eating utensils
- ☐ Drinking cup
- ☐ Pot grabber
- ☐ Soap/detergent
- ☐ Towel
- ☐ Plastic garbage bags
- ☐ Resealable plastic bags
- ☐ Water filter/purifier
- ☐ Water purification tablets
- ☐ Water bottle(s)
- ☐ Collapsible water container
- ☐ Lantern

References

1 American Red Cross. *Preparing for Events.* Available at: http://www.redcross
.org/portal/site/en/menuitem.d8aaecf214c576bf971e4cfe43181aa0/?vgnextoid
=46de1a53flc37110VgnVCM1000003481a10aRCRD&vgnextfmt=default.
Accessed February 7, 2009.

2. FEMA. *Are You Ready?* Available at: http://www.fema.gov/areyouready.
Accessed February 7, 2009.

3. Trip Resource. *International Travel Checklist.* Available at: http://www
.tripresource.com/beforeyougo.htm. Accessed February 7, 2009.

Risk Communication, Prevention, and the Media

Frederick J. Stoddard Jr., MD, Craig L. Katz, MD,
Edward M. Kantor, MD, Ann E. Norwood, MD,
and Joseph P. Merlino, MD, MPA

Your involvement in disaster response may occur close to home or across the globe. Let's return to our internist, Peter, introduced to you earlier in this volume. Peter sought to get the word out to the public in a variety of ways. Peter wanted to inform people as to what was occurring and where families, children, and others could go to find additional information or to receive medical care during a disaster, if necessary. Imagine that you are this internist and the disaster you are confronting is in your community. Walk for the moment in his shoes.

- Fear, confusion, and stigmatization are decreased by clear and consistent information.

- Communication about risk reduces the number of people inappropriately seeking medical help.

- Risk communication protects people from putting themselves in harm's way.

- Accurate positive communication increases the sense of control and mastery of the situation.

Definition

"Risk communication" is the term used by disaster response teams to describe effective communication during a crisis. The term encompasses exchange of information between individuals (e.g., you and your patients), groups (e.g., Peter and families in his community), and institutions (e.g., the local radio station broadcasting to the affected businesses and public institutions of the region).

Fear Lessened by Early, Accurate, Positive Information

Fear, confusion, and stigmatization can become major problems in disasters and are decreased by clear and consistent information.[1] Fears based on inaccurate information or mistaken understanding may result in large numbers of people seeking unnecessary medical help, which can overwhelm medical providers who are there for those truly in need of medical care (see Chapter 10, Medically Unexplained Symptoms). In addition, people could end up exposing themselves to unnecessary risks.

Most primary care clinicians not involved in disasters may give little thought to the importance of communication at times of disaster, how information is shared, and how it is best executed. Lessons learned from the major disasters and terrorist events over the last 15 years have led to the development of general guidelines for communicating during crises. Accurate and positive communication increases the sense of control and familiarity that people have about a disaster and its sequelae, increasing their mastery of the situation. As a clinician, you may provide reality-based reassurance to reduce anxiety, while also communicating about ongoing risks and safety. Whether in your practice or as a volunteer, during a disaster you play an important role in public communication about the nature of the risks, injuries, and deaths. Optimally, risk communication is planned before any disaster occurs and includes communication pre-event, at the time of and during the event, and post-event.[2] Pre-event communication is useful to deliver information aimed at lessening fear and encouraging confidence that the public will be protected. At the time of the event there is a need for clear, credible communication regarding the real risk and timely responses necessitated by the event. Post-event communication is useful to update information on the event, the success of interventions, and where to find help for those who continue to need it.

Mass Communication

In crafting a simple and clear message, it is best to present information about a specific subject or event, rather than multiple, lengthy, or conflicting messages.[2] Communication may be used to organize support through a variety of media venues including a statement transmitted by radio, web site, email, video, or poster. These should provide a realistic picture oriented at easing public concern. The message should describe how to reduce, risk, and provide guidance for how best to respond. Further resources should also be given for those wanting more information. Acknowledging uncertainty, which is often present in disasters, is part of the message.

In order to assist the relief agency, hospital, clinic, or other organization where you are working, it is helpful to participate in media interviews, broadcasts, or efforts at providing public information. Primary care providers working in collaboration with mental health professionals serve as important models for the delivery of effective risk communication and prevention for populations affected by disaster. It is essential to have a sense of what the public's understanding is prior to making statements and to accurately address or clarify that understanding. It is best to speak about those areas in which you as a clinician are comfortable and competent, sticking close to the known facts, while earnestly admitting what you are unsure about or do not know.

Media training is recommended in preparing to respond to disasters. It is helpful to practice prior to public speaking during a disaster, receiving feedback from someone knowledgeable about public communication.[3] Time allotted for media communication is limited, often reduced to only sound bites—your message should be concise, clear, and able to fit within a brief time frame. Use of positive or neutral terms is best because negative statements, even if accurate, may be misconstrued or heighten fear and anxiety. Empathic communication directed to those directly affected by the disaster, including media representatives who are often stressed themselves, is a core element of any media contact. Concluding any communications about disaster on a positive note is also helpful.[4,5]

Individual Communication

Even if you do not have contact with the media or large groups of people, it is useful to learn the basic principles used when speaking to the public so that you can effectively and reassuringly communicate in times of disaster.[6] Such principles may be applicable in your contact with individual patients amid catastrophe. In times of crisis, physicians and other health care providers are generally looked to as de facto leaders.

How you communicate with your patients on an individual level can contribute to the larger atmosphere of risk communications. This will especially be the case in situations where the public health has been threatened, as in biological terrorism. Here are some relevant principles:

1. *Listen to, acknowledge, and respect the fears, anxieties, and uncertainties of your patients. They want to know that you care before they care what you know.* After the tsunami, a woman who was terrified that she was about to die from the disaster was brought by her husband to the shelter. Reassurance had not relieved her fears so far. Although you could quickly examine her and tell her that she will be okay, it is more helpful to examine her, inquire what she is afraid of, explain that you can understand her being afraid, and tell her that her fears should lessen gradually in the days to come.

2. *Recognize that people are risk averse and when upset will often fixate on negatives. Be extremely careful in offering up these five "N" words—no, not, never, nothing, and none—and words with negative connotations.* Following a shipwreck, you unofficially hear that there are no survivors, and a concerned patient asks you if anyone has survived. Rather than stating that there are no survivors without official confirmation, it is best to convey your concern about those on board, while indicating that you do not have full information and hope that some have survived.

3. *Offer authentic statements of caring, empathy, and compassion while also taking time to listen, and back up your statements with actions.* In a follow-up visit, an elderly Arabic-speaking woman presents with her 2-year-old granddaughter who was burned. You speak to her through an interpreter, listening to her distress and praising her caring. You say you will help reduce the child's ongoing pain and suffering. If you have analgesics in appropriate dosage available, you can back up your statement with medication for the child. If you do not, it is better not to promise what you cannot provide.

4. *Be honest, ethical, frank, and open, recognizing that there are limits to what needs to be disclosed.* An example arises in instances where people inquire about fatalities. After 9/11, physicians with limited experience breaking bad news were repeatedly asked to tell loved ones about fatalities at emergency family centers in Manhattan.

Although families were desperate for information, it was necessary to be both supportive and honest in empathically disclosing established facts about a death, while, on the other hand, setting firm limits not to disclose unclear or hearsay information to grieving relatives. You also need to resist possible political pressure to prematurely release incomplete findings, as occurred after 9/11 when medical examiner staff was pressured to prematurely "finalize" reports on the remains of possible fire fighters and police officers.

5. *Avoid mixed or inconsistent verbal and non-verbal messages.* "Well, the hurricane may be over and help may be on the way, but maybe not" is an example of an unhelpful statement, even if true. It is more helpful to give an accurate statement, such as, "We're awaiting full information on the hurricane and are trying to obtain more medical help."

References

1. MacGregor DG, Fleming R. Risk perception and symptom reporting. *Risk Analysis*. 1996;16:773–783.

2. Beard R, Kantor E. *Managing the Message in Times of Crisis: Risk Communication and Mental Wellness in Disaster Health Care.* Charlottesville: University of Virginia Medical Reserve Corps; 2004.

3. Covello VT. *Lessons Learned From the Front Lines of Risk and Crisis Communication: 21 Guidelines for Effective Communication by Leaders Addressing High Anxiety, High Stress, or Threatening Situations.* Presented as part of keynote address at the U.S. Conference of Mayors Emergency, Safety, and Security Summit, Washington, DC; October 4, 2001.

4. Institute of Medicine. *Preparing for the Psychological Consequences of Terrorism: A Public Health Strategy.* Washington, DC: The National Academy of Sciences Institute of Medicine; 2003.

5. Norwood AH, Sermons WL, and Blumenfield M. *Crisis Communication: The Role of Psychiatric Leaders in Communicating with the Media and Government Officials at the Time of Disaster, Terrorism, and Other Crises.* Speaker-Elect Forum, American Psychiatric Association, Washington, DC; November 10, 2005.

6. SAMHSA. *Communicating in a Crisis: Risk Communication Guidelines for Public Officials 2002.* Available at: **http://www.riskcommunication.SAMHSA .gov.** Accessed March 17, 2009.

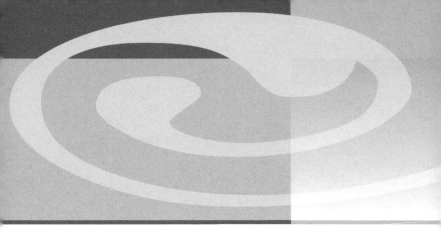

Assessment

Section Editor: Craig L. Katz, MD

Assessment: A Spectrum from Normal to Psychopathology

Craig L. Katz, MD

Following a memorial service at the former World Trade Center site in New York City just a month after the 9/11 terrorist attacks, family members returned to the Family Assistance Center in midtown Manhattan to collect urns with soil from "Ground Zero." The center was fully staffed, including an on-call medical team on which the internist, Peter, was volunteering. At one point, a worker from an agency involved in providing mass care for the families came running up to Peter and directed him to a woman who was sobbing soulfully while waiting in line for an urn. As she was doing so alongside of an attentive companion, Peter suggested there was no reason to intervene. She appeared to be displaying normal emotions under the circumstances. Peter chose instead to spend some time talking with the aid worker about how she was handling things.

- Reactions to disaster span the range of normal to abnormal.

- These include distress, behavior changes, and psychiatric disorder.

- Intensity, pervasiveness, and duration of reactions shape the need for clinical concern and intervention.

- Psychiatric symptoms also reflect the underlying personal meaning(s) of the event.

Understanding Human Reactions to Disaster

In 1957, a psychologist described human reaction to disasters as follows:

It is not easy to find out how disasters affect people. In the best of times our observations of human nature are rather rarely intensive or systematic. In the alarm, disorder, pain, and grief of large scale catastrophes, there have been too many urgent things to do.[1]

Human nature often defies cataloging, but it is fair to say we have come much further along in our understanding of disaster's psychological impact on people since this understatement.

A useful framework for understanding the psychological consequences of disasters encompasses three types of reactions—distress responses, changes in behavior, and diagnosed psychiatric illness (Figure 6.1).[2] Because some psychological consequences of disaster include positive reactions to the event, it might be more accurate to call these three areas "psychological consequences of potential concern" in your practice as a primary care clinician.

Distress responses of potential concern encompass changes in how people feel and think, and such responses may themselves be further separated into emotional, physical, and spiritual reactions. Emotional reactions are exemplified by the crying woman in the scenario after the memorial and can span a range of uncomfortable reactions including sadness, dysphoria, anxiety, and anger. Physical reactions can include medically unexplained physical symptoms or even panic-like symptoms such as palpitations or shortness of breath. Insomnia can also be a symptom. Cognitive reactions involve changes in how people think and can include confusion or forgetfulness. Spiritual reactions embrace

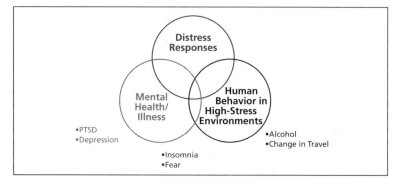

Figure 6.1   The psychological consequences of disasters span alterations in behavior, heightened distress, and, at the extreme, psychiatric disorders.

physical, emotional, and cognitive experiences influencing people's sense of security, integrity, meaning, and purpose.

Behavioral changes of potential concern reflect changes in how people do things and go about their lives (e.g., refusing to use air travel after 9/11). Of great concern would be behaviors such as alcohol or drug use or becoming more socially withdrawn.

A framework for thinking about psychiatric issues amid your medical work-up of disaster survivors is presented in Box 6.1.

Assessing the Severity of Peoples' Response to Disaster

There are several important points to make about the distress and behavioral reactions you may encounter in the patients you care for

Box 6.1 Effective Diagnosis—Guidelines for Including Psychiatric Considerations in Your Medical Work-ups Amid Disaster.[3–7]

Including behavioral and psychiatric considerations in your medical work-up increases the effectiveness of management because stress and trauma may contribute to your patients' physical complaints.

Psychiatric illness and behavioral contagion may overlap with medical manifestations of infectious, chemical, radioactive, or explosive injuries.

The order of assessment after physical trauma is:

1. Primary Survey (ATLS): ABCs (the greatest threats to life).

2. Secondary Survey (ATLS): Each part of body is examined.

3. Tertiary Survey—Psychiatric: The clinical interview identifies the most common psychiatric sequelae. Its elements are observation of appearance and behavior, level of consciousness, mental content, speech, orientation, memory, mood, and judgment.

   a. It may include the Mini-Mental State Examination (MMSE), which is brief and limited and may help identify patients with cognitive disturbance or dementia. It can also help identify sudden onset of cognitive problems together with altered consciousness, indicating that delirium is likely.

   b. The full clinical interview is required to identify dangerousness to self or others as well as other psychiatric symptoms requiring intervention.

after a disaster. First, many of these symptoms or behaviors are "normal" or adaptive in the acute aftermath of disaster, which can be defined as the days to weeks after a disaster occurs, perhaps lasting as long as 2 months.[8] The time frame in which these reactions occur is one way to help determine whether they are "normal" or "abnormal." For example, palpitations and anxiety are functional and even normative aspects of a so-called fight-or-flight reaction that enables someone to feel the need and have the capacity to flee from a burning building. Even if these experiences, especially anxiety, last for a few days after a catastrophic event, our level of clinical concern may not yet rise unless the symptoms are accompanied by physical complaints such as chest pain. When they last for weeks to months, into what we might call the post-acute phase, then their clinical significance as a mental health issue becomes more apparent.[9] Refusing to commute into London for a few days to a week after the 2005 terrorist attacks on that city's subway is understandable, especially as authorities work to assess and establish security, but doing so for weeks to months later, especially when a person's job is imperiled, should raise concerns.

Another dimension along which you may take the measure of distress or behavioral reactions to a disaster is the intensity of the reactions. Even if someone has suffered from anxiety for just a few days after a disaster, if that anxiety affects his functioning, then it has reached a level of clinical significance. For example, the anxious survivor may feel so distressed that he is not able to follow urgent recommendations made by the authorities regarding where to sleep, get provisions, or obtain medical care. People may lose their appetite to a degree that they become dehydrated or lose so much sleep that they can barely function at a time when maximal focus on one's own recovery efforts is essential.

At the most extreme end of functional impact are those people who become suicidal. It is natural for disaster survivors to pose newly burning spiritual questions about the meaning of life. It is also not uncommon or unusual for them to wish they could join or be with loved ones who have perished in the disaster. As discussed in greater detail in a later chapter, if this wish assumes a constancy or transforms into a plan of action to take one's life in order to join the dead, then you must institute an immediate clinical intervention. For instance, in the opening of this chapter, if the woman crying at the World Trade Center memorial was assessed and found to have suicidal wishes, you would need to provide further assessment and intervention.

Finally, you may also gauge the intensity of someone's distress or behavioral reactions to disasters by how much discomfort these things cause. This does not constitute an objective criterion for clinical concern. Yet it underscores how you can remind your patients that it is natural to be feeling badly but that no one should have to feel any more badly than necessary after disasters. Reminding your patients that what they feel is normal is an act of empathy that alone can help people to feel better. It is also an act of assessment that may open up necessary channels of psychological communication between you and your patient.

Discussion of distress and behavioral reactions to disaster as symptoms casts them as problems to be eradicated, much like you would approach a cough or a headache. However, too narrow of a focus on them as symptoms can overlook a complementary perspective—that which looks at symptoms as following common pathways to layers of personal meaning that lie underneath in the minds of survivors.[10] For example, although it is important to evaluate and treat trauma-related insomnia, the sleeplessness is also an opportunity to learn about what is on the mind of your patient. This can be accomplished by including a question like the following in your work-up: "What goes through your mind when you are lying awake at night?" Such inquiry, as with much of the process of assessment, has a psychotherapeutic as well as a diagnostic dimension.

Psychological studies have attempted to categorize the types of thoughts, rather than symptoms, people have in response to experiencing a disaster.[4] Thoughts may be about some of the following common themes: bewilderment; danger; impasse; desperation; apathy; helplessness; urgency; or discomfort. The bewildered person feels lost and overwhelmed whereas the person at an impasse feels stuck or paralyzed. You may gauge the clinical significance of such thinking much like a symptom—in terms of their intensity, pervasiveness, and duration. But, at the very least, they are also opportunities for you to learn more about the experiences of your patients.

At the most extreme end of human reactions is the third element of the triad of psychological consequences mentioned earlier: psychiatric disorders. The most common post-disaster psychiatric disorders are

PTSD, Major Depression, and alcohol use disorders, often seen in combination.[5] However, some conditions may combine elements of PTSD-like anxiety symptoms and depressive symptoms. These disorders can be broadly conceptualized as syndromes, or amalgams of symptoms (e.g., distress or behavioral reactions) that have lasted too long and with too much intensity. With the passage from the acute phase to the post-acute phase of disasters, persistent symptoms may coalesce into disorders.[6] For example, PTSD can be thought of, both biologically and experientially, as a flight-or-fight reaction that has outlived its initial utility. The person is acting as though there is something to flee or fear when no such thing exists anymore. Whereas symptoms may be treated and psychological reactions should be explored, once disorders occur, they should be treated, either by you or a mental health colleague if available, or together in collaborative care (e.g., telepsychiatry).

Conclusion

The tears of the woman at the 9/11 memorial service in the opening example likely represent a normal expression of distress. A number of elements can guide you as a primary care professional in assessing the severity of her distress. Concern should be heightened if she reports that she cries all of the time in a way that feels either excessive or limiting. Even if the woman has no other psychological manifestations of concern, the burden she is feeling because of her sadness may raise it to the level of clinical concern and invite the prescription of help of various kinds. Or, if she indeed has other symptoms, such as loss of motivation to go about her life or insomnia, then consideration needs to be given to the possibility that she is developing a psychiatric disorder requiring very specific interventions. No matter what, if she were alone, it would be compassionate for you to approach her and ask if there is anything you can do for her.

References

1. Wolfenstein M. *Disaster: A Psychological Essay.* Chicago: The Free Press; 1957.

2. Ursano RJ. *Terrorism and Mental Health: Public Health and Primary Care.* Presentation at the Eighteenth Annual Rosalyn Carter Symposium on Mental Health Policy. Status Report: *Meeting the Mental Health Needs of the Country in the Wake of September 11, 2001.* The Carter Center, Atlanta; November 2002.

3. Rundell JR. A consultation liaison psychiatry approach to disaster/terrorism victim assessment and management. In: Ursano RJ, Fullerton CS, Norwood AE, Eds. *Terrorism and Disaster: Individual and Community Mental Health Interventions.* New York: Cambridge University Press; 2003:107–120.

4. Rundell JR, Christopher GW. Differentiating manifestations of infection from psychiatric disorders and fears of having been exposed to bioterrorism. In: Ursano RJ, Norwood AE, Fullerton CS, Eds. *Bioterrorism: Psychological and Public Health Interventions.* Cambridge: Cambridge University Press; 2004:88–108.

5. Pastel RH, Ritchie EC. Mitigation of psychological effects of weapons of mass destruction. In: Ritchie EC, Watson PJ, Friedman MJ, Eds. *Interventions Following Mass Violence and Disasters: Strategies for Mental Health Practice.* New York: The Guilford Press; 2006:300–318.

6. American College of Surgeons. Advance trauma life support. Initial assessment and management. In: *Advanced Trauma Life Support for Doctors: Student Course Manual.* Chicago: American College of Surgeons; 1997.

7. Folstein MF, Folstein SE, McHugh PR. Mini-Mental State: a practical method for grading the cognitive state of patients for the clinician. *J Psychiatr Res.* 1975;12:189–198.

8. Katz CL, Pellegrino L, Pandya A, Ng A, DeLisi L. Research on psychiatric outcomes subsequent to disasters: a review of the literature. *Psychiat Res.* 2002;110(3):201–217.

9. Disaster Psychiatry Outreach. (2008). *The Essentials of Disaster Psychiatry: A Training Course for Mental Health Professionals.* New Caanan, CT: Unpublished manuscript.

10. Katz CL, Nathaniel R. Disasters, psychiatry, and psychodynamics. *J Am Acad Psychoanal.* 2002;30(4):519–530.

Assessment and Management of Suicide After Disasters

Erick Hung, MD

Following a hurricane, Peter approaches a 24-year-old woman in the emergency shelter who is crying at her bed. The woman was just informed that her mother passed away in the hurricane. The woman appears distraught and volunteers, "I wish I were with my mother."

Several weeks later, a 54-year-old man who lost his house and family in the disaster makes a medical appointment with Peter in the clinic. During the clinic visit, the man tells Peter that he has not been sleeping or eating, and is having more frequent thoughts of death. Peter asks the man if he has any guns at home, and he replies, "Yes, I am so ashamed to say this but sometimes I hold the gun and think of just ending it all."

- Passive and active thoughts of death as well as suicidal ideation can be a common reaction following a disaster and need to be closely monitored and discussed.

- Know the important risk factors as well as the protective factors for suicide.

- Provide a framework for assessing an individual's risk for suicide.

- Know your resources and how you will manage individuals at moderate to high risk of suicide.

Introduction

In the aftermath of a disaster, acute stress, bereavement, property loss, and the disruption of social networks can potentially lead to mental health problems, including depression, hopelessness, anger, and aggression. Although it is a normal and common reaction for disaster victims to feel angry at the losses that they face, feel helpless, or even transiently feel as if life is not worth living, for some individuals, these thoughts and feelings may lead to potentially self-injurious or violent behavior.[1] Suicide is thankfully a rare event under normal circumstances, and the empirical data available on suicide in relation to disasters, such as following the 9/11 terrorist attacks and Hurricane Katrina, are mixed.[2–7] Indeed, in only one study has it been clearly shown that suicidality increases after disasters—here the prevalence of suicidal ideation increased from 2.8% to 6.4% following Hurricane Katrina, and suicide plans increased from 1% to 2.5%.[8]

With destruction and death all around the scene of a disaster, it is to be expected that issues about the meaning and value of life will arise for survivors. In some cases, these issues will take the form of suicidality. For all of these reasons, clinicians like Peter should be prepared to address questions of suicidality much more than in their usual practice. Suicidality necessitates an assessment for safety while also affording a window into a patient's distress.

Suicide Risk Assessment: Risk Factors and Protective Factors

What makes suicide risk assessment difficult in a disaster is that clinicians must provide not only reassurance and normalize common reactions to the disaster, but they must also remain vigilant in monitoring for active suicidal thoughts and feelings. Passive suicidal thoughts (e.g., general thoughts and feelings about wanting to be dead or about taking one's life that may transiently pass through a victim's mind) require further inquiry but may necessitate only reassurance and further monitoring. Active suicidal thoughts (e.g., specific thoughts about ending one's life in the immediate future) require more intensive evaluation and could possibly involve mental health professionals and involuntarily detaining someone to protect them. Distinguishing between passive and active suicidal ideation, a crucial decision point in assessment, is not straightforward. Clinicians are not very good at predicting suicide.[9] Although an understanding of risk factors and protective factors allows clinicians to recognize individuals at relatively increased risk for suicide, it does not allow for accurate prediction.

Some important risk factors include a past history of suicide attempts, active suicidal ideation with a specific intent and plan, access to weapons, acute intoxication or ongoing substance use, acute anxiety, and psychotic thinking. Some protective factors include positive social support, positive coping skills, and a sense of responsibility to family.[10]

Suicide Risk Assessment: Providing a Framework

The list of suicide risk and protective factors is exhaustive and often difficult to use in clinical encounters. Assessment involves combining an analysis of a patient's risk factors and protective factors with information about the patient's suicidal ideation and planning. Several strategies for organizing information in your assessment have been developed. Here are two helpful mnemonics (see Box 7.1).

Regardless of your preferences for organizing information, as a clinician assessing suicide risk in the aftermath of a disaster it is essential that you ultimately estimate a patient's suicide risk. Wherever possible, we recommend estimating a victim's suicide risk in this basic framework: low imminent risk for suicide, moderate imminent risk for suicide, and high imminent risk for suicide. Here is a framework for organizing your approach to suicidality (see Table 7.1).

There are no exact algorithms for assignment of risk. In general, the more risk factors present, the higher the risk. And active suicidal thoughts, a past history of suicidality, and presence of substance use should likely be given much greater weight than other risk factors.

Box 7.1 Helpful Mnemonics to Organize Risk Factors for Suicide

Sad Persons	No Hope
Sex	No framework for meaning
Age	Overt change in clinical condition
Depression	Hostile interpersonal environment
Previous attempt	Out of hospital recently
Ethanol abuse	Predisposing personality factors
Rational thought loss	Excuses for dying to help others
Social supports lacking	
Organized plan	
No spouse	
Sickness	

Table 7.1 Chronologic Framework for Approaching Suicide. The first three columns represent factors that contribute to the assessment of suicide risk (column 4) and resulting intervention (column 5).

Historical Factors (Past)	Clinical Factors (Present)	Situational Factors (Future)	Summary Judgment of Imminent Risk for Suicide	Interventions
			☐ High Risk ☐ Moderate Risk ☐ Low Risk	

Once you have placed a disaster survivor in one of these three categories (low, moderate, or high imminent risk), your specific interventions, either at the disaster site or in the office, clinic, or hospital, will be guided based on the acuity level (see Management of Suicidality, on page 58).

Suicide Risk Assessment: Helpful Interview Techniques and Clinical Rating Scales

Many clinicians avoid talking about suicide because of a common myth that talking about suicide will put the idea of suicide into an individual's mind.[9] Not only is it alright to talk about suicide, it is imperative that you do so. Such a discussion has the potential of saving a life or at least providing the relief of unburdening oneself of such thoughts. Table 7.2 lists some basic suicide questions to ask when you suspect an elevated suicide risk in an individual.

Talking about death and suicide is extremely difficult. Individuals are often ambivalent, reluctant, defensive, cautious, stigmatized, overwhelmed, and disturbed by suicidal thoughts, intentions, and plans. Consequently, accurately eliciting these thoughts and feelings is challenging.[9] Direct questions sometimes need to be re-asked in different ways to elicit accurate information. Cultural and religious taboos, and the need to use interpreters, may also make eliciting accurate information challenging.

Even with the best of interviewing techniques, at the end of your encounter with the patient, you may still feel uncertain or confused.

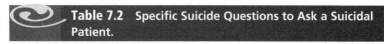

Table 7.2 Specific Suicide Questions to Ask a Suicidal Patient.

Questions to Ask

✓ Does the person have intent?
✓ Does the person have a plan? If so, have the person describe the plan.
✓ Does the person have a target? Self or others?
✓ Does the individual have the means? Access to weapons?
✓ Does the person have prior risk history? If so, how serious and under what circumstances?
✓ What sort of losses or injuries did the person sustain after the disaster?
✓ Is the patient intoxicated?
✓ Is the patient acutely psychotic (e.g., hearing voices, talking to himself, rambling about paranoid themes, including doomsday, conspiracies, etc.)?
✓ Is the patient dazed, or in a state of dissociation, wandering, confused, purposeless activity, refusing food or shelter?
✓ Is the patient having uncontrolled panic? Complaining of heart palpitations, shortness of breath without medical causes?
✓ Is the patient maintaining nutrition and hydration?
✓ What level of support, perceived vs. real, does the individual have, in light of the disaster?
✓ Are there any appropriate coping skills and support that can be encouraged and reinforced?
✓ What safety plan can be instituted and accepted by the person?

Obtaining collateral information is extremely helpful in these circumstances and is an accepted part of the work done by mental health professionals. Other individuals who know the patient may have invaluable information that will assist you in your suicide risk assessment. Remember that the context of your assessment is an emergency situation and thereby usually constitutes an exception to confidentiality and informed consent.[11] If you are uncertain in your assessment, consult a mental health professional if possible. Most importantly, trust your gut instinct.

In addition to direct interviewing, clinical rating scales are becoming more common in the assessment of suicide risk. Although these rating scales are not meant to be a substitute for a clinical assessment and direct interviewing, they may have some utility in screening large volumes of patients so that you can prioritize which individuals to interview further in your disaster triage assessment.[12–14]

Management of Suicidality

If your summary judgment of an individual's imminent risk for suicide is low, then you may not need to make any further interventions on this matter. If your summary judgment of an individual's imminent risk for suicide is moderate or high, it is essential that you consult with or refer to a mental health professional at the disaster site (psychiatrist, psychologist, licensed social worker). In the event that a mental health professional is not available either on-site or via telepsychiatry, consider the following:

Moderate Acute Suicide Risk

- Are there any active behavioral symptoms (anxiety, psychosis, depression) that would benefit acutely from psychotropic medications? Remember, meds take time to work, so you need to ensure the patient's safety in the meantime.
- How can I increase the individual's current level of psychosocial support?
- Are there other individuals who can monitor this victim's level of safety in a medically unsupervised setting?
- Is the patient intoxicated? Being intoxicated increases suicide risk, and the individual may require intervention.
- Can I remove any potential lethal means? Remove guns at home? Remove lethal medications? Remove the patient from the current setting?

High Acute Suicide Risk

- Do I need to call the police in order to detain this individual to protect her own safety (e.g., civil or involuntary commitment)?
- Does this individual meet the involuntary commitment requirements in my particular area (differs from state to state)?
- If involuntary commitment requirements are met, under whose authority can I place this individual on an involuntary legal hold?

In disaster relief work, if mental health professionals are not directly available for on-site consultation for individuals with moderate to high imminent suicide risks, a consultation can be done over the phone with a mental health professional in a central command office. Know your resources for high suicide risk individuals before making your initial assessment. This will facilitate and expedite your management. Assessment of suicidal ideation or intent is a life-saving intervention.

References

1. Solomon SD. Mental health effects of natural and human-made disasters. *PTSD Res Q.* 1992;3(1):1–7.

2. Somasundaram DJ, Rajadurai S. War and suicide in Northern Sri Lanka. *Acta Psychiatr Scand.* 1995;91:1–4.

3. Lester D. The effect of war on suicide rates: a study of France from 1826 to 1913. *Eur Arch Psychiatry Clin Neurosci.* 1993;242:248–249.

4. Krug EG, et al. Suicide after natural disasters. *N Engl J Med.* 1998; 338(6):373–378.

5. Kucerova H. Reaction of patients in the psychiatric out-patient department to floods in 1997. *Ceska a Slovenka Psychiatre.* 1999;95(7):476–482.

6. Shiori T, et al. The Kobe earthquake and reduced suicide rate in Japanese males. *Archives of General Psychiatry.* 1999;56(3):282–283.

7. Voracek M, Sonneck G. Suicide after natural disasters and statistical disasters: a comment. *Archives of Suicide Research.* 2002;6(4):399–401.

8. Kessler RC, et al. Trends in mental illness and suicidality after Hurricane Katrina. *Molecular Psychiatry.* 2008;13:374–384.

9. Shea SC. *The Practical Art of Suicide Assessment: A Guide to Mental Health Professionals and Substance Abuse Counselors.* New York: John Wiley & Sons, Inc.; 1999.

10. American Psychiatric Association. Practice guideline for the assessment and treatment of patients with suicidal behaviors. *Am J Psychiatry.* 2003;160(11).

11. Borak J, Veilleux S. Informed consent in emergency settings. *Ann Emerg Med.* 1984;13(9):731–735.

12. Cochrane-Brink KA, et al. Clinical rating scales in suicide risk assessment. *General Hospital Psychiatry.* 2000;22:445–451.

13. Range LM, Knott EC. Twenty suicide assessment instruments: evaluation and recommendations. *Death Stud.* 1997;21:25–58.

14. Hockberger RS, Rothstein RJ. Assessment of suicide potential by nonpsychiatrists using the SAD PERSONS score. *J Emerg Med.* 1988;6:99–107.

Screening for Mental Health Issues Following Disaster

Kristina Jones, MD

After 9/11, Ben, a construction worker laborer in his 40s, worked for 6 months at the Ground Zero site. When he presented to a physician with complaints of eye irritation, he appeared fatigued and thin, and incidentally mentioned that he had been unable to sleep for over a month since finishing his work at the site. He was prescribed sleeping pills for his insomnia. At that time, the physician told Ben that it was normal to be upset and physically exhausted given what he had seen and done. Unfortunately, he was not questioned about his alcohol or drug use. Ben was, in fact, a patient with 8 years of sobriety from alcohol and heroin, and he had relapsed on alcohol following the funeral of a friend who died in the 9/11 terrorist attacks. Previously, Ben's drinking had led him to a heroin relapse lasting several months, which required detox. Ben's loss of sobriety was a direct result of his exposure to traumatic material encountered at the site and bereavement following the disaster.

- A primary care clinician's screening during the impact phase of a disaster should include psychiatric symptoms and reflect vigilance for presentations of severe disturbances.

- Formal psychiatric assessments may take place in the acute and post-acute phases of disaster.

- Both child and adult screening tools are available to detect distress of clinical significance and common post-disaster diagnoses such as post-traumatic stress disorder (PTSD), major depression, and alcohol abuse/dependence.

Introduction

A brief screening for alcohol or drug abuse might have mitigated Ben's relapse. Despite your many responsibilities as a primary care clinician in the aftermath of disaster, there are ways to efficiently screen for mental health problems, including general psychiatric assessment, suicidality, medically unexplained symptoms, and bereavement. Assessment of psychological reactions to disaster includes emotional, cognitive, behavioral, and physical dimensions. Specific strategies apply to each stage after the disaster. This timeline was reviewed in Chapter 6, Assessment: A Spectrum from Normal to Psychopathology, and is summarized in Table 8.1.

Impact Phase: 0 to 48 Hours After the Event

The emotional and behavioral reactions characteristic of the impact phase may be quite dramatic but in this early phase are expected to be brief, transient, and fluid. During the first 48 hours, psychiatric assessment is not only impractical but also likely to yield many false positives. Focus instead on the key issues in Table 8.2, and invite the patient to return for re-evaluation after initial triage, with or without intervention.

Acute Phase and Post-Acute Phase: Weeks to Months to Years Later

As the days give way to weeks and months and beyond, you can begin to conduct a standard mental health assessment using a conventional psychiatric interview format. The Disaster-Specific Mental Health Assessment Interview, shown in Table 8.3, includes disaster-specific items and assumes that you have completed the other parts of the medical assessment.

Common Diagnoses After Disaster

The Disaster-Specific Mental Health Assessment Interview (Table 8.3) will reveal the most common post-disaster diagnoses, which include

 Table 8.1   **Stages of Disaster**

Impact Phase:	0–48 hours after the event
Acute Phase:	1–8 weeks after the event
Post-Acute Phase:	Approximately 2 months after the event and beyond

Table 8.2 Impact Phase Assessment

Key Points

✓ Is the patient suicidal?
✓ Is the patient intoxicated?
✓ Is the patient homicidal or inappropriately armed in defense against feared attack?
✓ Is the patient acutely psychotic (hearing voices, talking to himself, rambling about paranoid themes, including doomsday, conspiracies, etc.)?
✓ Is the patient dazed, or in a state of dissociation, wandering, confused, pursuing purposeless activity, or refusing food or shelter?
✓ Is the patient having uncontrolled panic? Complaining of heart palpitations, shortness of breath without medical causes?
✓ Is the patient maintaining hydration and nutrition?

major depression, alcohol abuse/dependence, and anxiety disorders such as post-traumatic stress disorder, panic disorder, or generalized anxiety disorder. It is possible to screen for these conditions in large numbers of patients with relative efficiency. Screening is especially important for patients with known risk factors for post-disaster psychiatric sequelae, including high exposure to the event, prior psychiatric history, prior trauma, pre-disaster psychosocial problems, and loss of social support in the aftermath of the disaster. The Patient Health Questionnaire (PHQ) is a useful tool for conducting screenings.[1] Patients are

 Table 8.3 Disaster-Specific Mental Health Assessment

• **Identifying Data:** Age, gender, occupational status, social supports, and housing status
• **Chief Complaint/History of the Presenting Symptoms**
• **Review of Symptoms (including but not limited to):** Anxiety, panic, insomnia, loss of appetite, dissociation, depression, grief, mania, suicidality, homicidality, and access to weapons, or carrying of weapons, psychosis, paranoia, and functioning in daily life
• **Psychiatric History:** Pre-disaster medications and prior traumas
• **Substance Abuse**
• **Pre-Disaster Social History:** Patient's connection to nuclear family, extended family, social network, work, and financial status
• **Additional Items Associated with Disaster:** Need for, and access to, temporary shelter, food, emergency benefits, childcare, communications with family and friends, faith community, or pastoral counseling

responsible for completing the form (available in both English and Spanish), and therefore they must be able to read and comprehend it.

The PHQ provides a brief comprehensive screening for a number of disorders associated with disasters, specifically major depression, alcohol abuse disorder, panic disorder, and generalized anxiety disorder but not PTSD. After a disaster, these disorders are diagnosed and treated the same way they would be in a non-disaster situation when the resources are available. It is important to treat symptoms promptly and not to minimize them as a normal reaction to disaster, particularly when the acute phase gives way to the post-acute phase, at which point the vast majority of people should have made a significant recovery and resumed ordinary social, familial, or occupational duties. In addition to developing the preceding disorders, approximately 7% to 12% of those exposed to a disaster may develop post-traumatic stress disorder, for which a different screening tool is commonly used.[2,3]

Post-Traumatic Stress Disorder

As the one post-disaster diagnosis that is trauma-specific and therefore least likely to be familiar to you, post-traumatic stress disorder deserves further explanation. PTSD is an anxiety disorder that includes exposure to a traumatic event in which the person experienced, witnessed, or was confronted with actual or threatened death, serious injury, or physical harm to the integrity of self or others, and the person's response involved intense fear, helplessness, or horror.[4] Following this experience and response, the patient develops symptoms in three separate domains: re-experiencing, avoidance, and hyper-arousal.

The patient must have at least one re-experiencing symptom, which include intrusive distressing recollections of the event (in children, repetitive play may occur in which themes or aspects of the trauma are expressed), recurrent nightmares, flashbacks, physical reactivity upon reminders, and intense psychological distress upon reminders.

Furthermore, the patient must have three or more avoidant symptoms, which include efforts to avoid feelings, thoughts, or conversations about the trauma; avoidance of people, places, or things that arouse recollections of the trauma; difficulty remembering details of the trauma; diminished interest in activities; feelings of detachment from others; restricted affect; and sense of a foreshortened life span.

Finally, the patient must have at least two symptoms of increased arousal, as indicated by insomnia, irritability or anger, hyper-vigilance, and exaggerated startle response.

It is critical for the medical professional to be aware that many patients may have a few of these symptoms and, although not meeting full criteria for PTSD, may have clinically significant partial PTSD.

Many patients will be familiar with terms like *shell shock* and *trauma*. Some patients will announce that they are "highly traumatized" or they will declare that they have PTSD because in U.S. popular culture, the term is often used as a synonym for shock or distress. You should conduct a formal assessment when there is reason to believe your patient might have PTSD. A useful tool in the disaster setting is the Primary Care PTSD Screen (Table 8.4), which was developed by the National Center for PTSD.[3]

Since the Primary Care PTSD Screen is not available in Spanish, an alternative questionnaire used extensively in research and clinical settings

 Table 8.4   Primary Care PTSD Screen

In your life, have you ever had any experience that was so frightening, horrible, or upsetting that, *in the past month,* you...

1. **Have had nightmares about it or thought about it when you did not want to?**

    YES   NO

2. **Tried hard not to think about it or went out of your way to avoid situations that reminded you of it?**

    YES   NO

3. **Were constantly on guard, watchful, or easily startled?**

    YES   NO

4. **Felt numb or detached from others, activities, or your surroundings?**

    YES   NO

Current research suggests that the results of the primary care PTSD should be considered "positive" if a patient answers "yes" to any three (3) items.

A positive response to the screen does not necessarily indicate that a patient has PTSD. However, a positive response does indicate that a patient may have PTSD or trauma-related problems, and further investigation of trauma symptoms by a mental health professional may be warranted.

is the PTSD Symptom Checklist, which has 17 questions.[5] The PTSD Symptom Checklist is also available in a short form, with only six questions.[6] Both versions are relatively simple to complete.

Children

After a disaster, one of the most common mental health questions asked of health care providers is what constitutes "normal" reactions for children. Anxious parents should be referred to child social work and mental health professionals for guidance. In the initial stage, try to have available patient handouts that explain children's frequent reactions, which you can give to the parents. These handouts are available through the American Academy of Child and Adolescent Psychiatry at **www.aacap.org**. For more on screening for PTSD symptoms in children, see Chapter 9. Children who come to clinical attention via parents or teachers can be screened using the Pediatric Symptom Checklist (PSC), reproduced on page 72.[7] This is a broad-ranging checklist of behaviors designed to alert physicians to common pediatric presentations of anxiety, depression, and trauma. The PSC is especially useful because it is administered by parents, available in a range of languages, and because it has been validated and found to be highly specific. Of the children who are negative on the PSC screen for behavioral disturbance, 95% will be identified as unimpaired when a full evaluation is performed by a qualified pediatric mental health specialist. The efficacy of the PSC screen enables pediatric mental health specialists to provide children with effective treatment.

Conclusion

Assessment during impact phase of a disaster should focus on psychiatric symptoms, while being vigilant for presentations of severe psychiatric syndromes such as panic disorder or psychosis. A complete formal psychiatric assessment can be deferred until the acute or post-acute phases of disaster. Screening tools that can detect common post-disaster diagnoses such at PTSD, major depression, and alcohol or substance abuse are available for children and for adults.

References

1. Patient Health Questionnaire Screener. 2008. Available at: **http://www.phqscreeners.com/overview.aspx#**. Accessed May 18, 2008.

2. Perrin M, DiGrande L, Wheeler K, Thorpe L, Farfel M, Brackbill R. Differences in PTSD prevalence and associated risk factors among World Trade Center disaster rescue and recovery workers. *Am J Psychiatry.* 2007; 164(9):1385–1394.

3. National Center for Post-Traumatic Stress Disorder. Primary Care PTSD Screen. 2007. Available at: **http://www.ncptsd.va.gov/ncmain/ncdocs/fact_shts/fs_screen_disaster.html**. Accessed February 21, 2009.

4. American Psychiatric Association. *Diagnostic and Statistical Manual of Mental Disorders.* 4th ed. Washington, DC: American Psychiatric Association; 2000.

5. National Center for Post-Traumatic Stress Disorder. Post-Traumatic Stress Disorder Symptom Checklist (Spanish and English). 2008. Available at: **http://www.ncptsd.va.gov/ncmain/ncdocs/assmnts/ptsd_checklist_pcl.html**. Accessed February 21, 2009.

6. National Center for Post-Traumatic Stress Disorder. Post-Traumatic Stress Disorder Symptom Checklist, Short Form. 2007. Available at: **http://www.ncptsd.va.gov/ncmain/ncdocs/assmnts/short_form_of_the_ptsd_checklistcivilian_version.html**. Accessed February 21, 2009.

7. Department of Child Psychiatry, Massachusetts General Hospital. Pediatric Symptom Checklist. 2008. Available at: **http://www2.massgeneral.org/allpsych/pediatricsymptomchecklist/psc_home.htm**. Accessed February 21, 2009.

Children and Families

Frederick J. Stoddard Jr., MD
Todd F. Holzman, MD

In the book's Introduction, the priest raises a concern about the impact of air raids on the children of his community in Sri Lanka. Ann, a pediatrician who volunteered for a relief team, sees a 13-year-old girl, Lakshmi, who has been very fearful for 2 months to leave home and return to school, as her classmates have done. Lakshmi's father was injured in the air raids and has been unable to return to work. Her pregnant mother (and the whole family) is grieving her own father's death while trying to provide for her family of eight children, including an 11-month-old, 2-year-old, and 3½-year-old. Ann wonders how she can be of most help.

Ann considers several questions. Are they safe? Do they have food and shelter? The first concern in assessing a situation like Lakshmi's is safety. In the context of major disasters and political conflicts many children and families are refugees and at great risk, possibly for many years.[1,2] When a child is injured, his or her emotional and psychological risk is made even greater from pain, stress, and depression.[3] Is the family in danger, either from further bombing, from

- Basic questions to ask with regard to children: Are they safe? Do they have food and shelter? Have they suffered prior trauma?

- Young children are especially vulnerable to the effects of separation, abandonment, and parental impairment, illness, or death.

- Infants, toddlers, school age children, and adolescents may be differentially reactive to stress related to their developmental stages.

- In assessing the factors strengthening families' resiliency, it is critical to consider their extended family, school and occupational supports, economic resources, religious affiliations, and ethnic and community ties.

damage to their home, the injuries to caretakers, or from hunger or disease? Are the young children adequately nourished and cared for? Have brothers, sisters, parents, or relatives been killed, injured, or are they missing? Is the fate of relatives or friends unknown? Relief organizations such as the International Red Cross provide initial food and shelter after disasters to affected families, but if the community is very remote, if there is extensive community damage, or if political factors prevent relief efforts, there can be delays in reaching everyone who is most affected.

Clinical Assessment

Once safety is assured, Ann can conduct a more traditional clinical assessment on Lakshmi. Since it is likely that a family member has brought her to Ann, the assessment ideally should be done in part with a family member present and in part with the child alone; however, this may not be possible. Family members may minimize children's reactions, especially when they themselves are impacted. Ann may be depending on a family member as an interpreter, and, although potentially necessary under the circumstances, this is not optimal as this sibling or other relative is likely to have intense, personal emotional reactions and little training for disaster response. Family members may tend to interpret answers to questions differently from what is actually said by the patient. In assessing Lakshmi's apparent phobic response about returning to school, screening questions may help (see Chapter 8, Screening for Mental Health Issues Following Disaster).

Ann can first assess the extent of the problem. Did any bombing occur near the school, thereby giving some reality to Lakshmi's degree of fearfulness? Or is the fear more a fear of leaving home during a frightening time? Has Lakshmi been avoiding school? Has she had other school problems before this? Or is she wishing she could return to school? Has she given up her usual play activities? Is she sleeping well? Has Lakshmi had other post-traumatic symptoms since the bombing, such as re-experiencing, nightmares, hyper-arousal, or increased startle? In her mother's opinion, what has helped or made things worse?

Ann also should consider factors that may be contributing to Lakshmi's condition. How much is her pregnant mother depending on her to help with the younger children? Has Lakshmi experienced prior trauma, such as an injury, or been physically or sexually abused? Could she be pregnant? Have the health needs of her injured father or pregnant mother been evaluated and attended to? Are there members of Lakshmi's extended family or friends nearby who could be of assistance to her family? Can the priest's parish provide any assistance to help Lakshmi, her grieving mother, and their family? These are just some of the important questions to consider in assessing Lakshmi's fear of returning to school and how best to help her and her family.[4,5] The evidence base for understanding children's responses to disasters is in an early phase, although it is expanding gradually.

Developmental Responses to Disaster: Infants, Children, and Adolescents

Infants, children, and adolescents will respond to disasters with the developmental skills they have achieved. Loss of recently acquired skills may be the most telling signs of difficulty coping with the disaster, especially for young children. Thus, the child may not be where she should be behaviorally, socially, and psychologically.

Infants and toddlers are entirely dependent on their caretakers, and the primary care clinician is often very experienced in assessing and intervening with problems in this age group, especially as problems relate to matters of nutrition and illness. Mental health issues such as maternal-infant stress, anxiety, phobias, withdrawal or depression, sleeping or eating problems, or refusal to play may be more subtle and discovered only when specifically asked about. Sometimes a child with intellectual or cognitive impairment may mistakenly be thought to have a physical or emotional illness. Help in recognizing such issues is possible with screening tools, such as the Pediatric Symptom Checklist (Table 9.1) where a score of 28 or higher indicates the child may be at risk, or the Child Stress Disorder Checklist (Table 9.2). An example might be Lakshmi's 3½-year-old sister, Tanya, who is very close to Lakshmi and came along to the consultation with Ann. Tanya appeared very clingy and withdrawn and possibly undernourished. When Ann asked her mother if she was worried about Tanya, her mother said that Tanya changed after her father came home injured, seemed more frightened of strangers, and wouldn't leave her

Table 9.1   Pediatric Symptom Checklist (PSC) for Screening for Psychiatric Disorders in Children

DATE _____
COMPLETED BY _____

NAME_____
RECORD # _____
D.O.B._____
USE IMPRINTER HERE

Pediatric Symptom Checklist (PSC)

Emotional and physical health go together in children. Because parents are often the first to notice a problem with their child's behavior, emotions or learning, you may help your child get the best care possible by answering these questions. Please indicate which statement best describes your child.

Please mark under the heading that best describes your child:

		NEVER (0)	SOMETIMES (1)	OFTEN (2)
1. Complains of aches and pains	1.			
2. Spends more time alone	2.			
3. Tires easily, has little energy	3.			
4. Fidgety, unable to sit still	4.			
5. Has trouble with teacher	5.			
6. Less interested in school	6.			
7. Acts as if driven by a motor	7.			
8. Daydreams too much	8.			
9. Distracted easily	9.			
10. Is afraid of new situations	10.			
11. Feels sad, unhappy	11.			
12. Is irritable, angry	12.			
13. Feels hopeless	13.			
14. Has trouble concentrating	14.			
15. Less interested in friends	15.			
16. Fights with other children	16.			
17. Absent from school	17.			
18. School grades dropping	18.			
19. Is down on him or herself	19.			
20. Visits the doctor with doctor finding nothing wrong	20.			
21. Has trouble sleeping	21.			
22. Worries a lot	22.			
23. Wants to be with you more than before	23.			
24. Feels he or she is bad	24.			
25. Takes unnecessary risks	25.			
26. Gets hurt frequently	26.			
27. Seems to be having less fun	27.			
28. Acts younger than children his or her age	28.			
29. Does not listen to rules	29.			
30. Does not show feelings	30.			
31. Does not understand other people's feelings	31.			
32. Teases others	32.			
33. Blames others for his or her troubles	33.			
34. Takes things that do not belong to him or her	34.			
35. Refuses to share	35.			

Total score _____

Does your child have any emotional or behavioral problems for which she/he needs help? __No __Yes
Are there any services that you would like your child to receive for these problems?   __No __Yes

If yes, what type of services? _____

Source: ©Jellinek MS, Murphy JM. Massachusetts General Hospital.
English PSC Gouverneur. Available at: **http://psc.partners.org**. Accessed March 17, 2009.

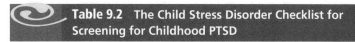

Table 9.2 The Child Stress Disorder Checklist for Screening for Childhood PTSD

Child Stress Disorder Checklist
(v. 3.0 3/07)

Child's Name (or ID#): _____ Age: ___ Sex: M F
Person Completing Questionnaire: _____ Date: _____
Relationship to Child: _____

Has your child experienced or witnessed an event that caused or threatened to cause serious harm to him or herself or to someone else? Please check any and all events and age(s) of your child at the time of the events below.

1. Car accident: _____ Age(s) _____   5. Physical Illness: _____ Age(s) _____
2. Other accident: _____ Age(s) _____   6. Physical Assault: _____ Age(s) _____
3. Fire: _____ Age(s) _____   7. Sexual Assault: _____ Age(s) _____
4. Storm: _____ Age(s) _____   8. Any Other Event: _____ Age(s) _____

Directions: Below is a list of behaviors that describe reactions that children may have following a frightening event. For each item that describes your child **NOW** or **WITHIN THE PAST MONTH**, please circle 2 if the item is **VERY TRUE** or **OFTEN TRUE** of your child. Circle 1 if the item is **SOMEWHAT** or **SOMETIMES TRUE** of your child. If the item is **NOT TRUE** of your child, circle 0. Please answer all items as well as you can, even if some do not seem to apply to your child. The term "event" refers to the **most** stressful experience you have described above.

0 1 2   Child reports more physical complaints when reminded of the event, such as headaches, stomachaches, nausea, difficulty breathing.

0 1 2   Child reports that he or she does not want to talk about the event.

0 1 2   Child startles easily. For example, he or she jumps when hears sudden or loud noises.

0 1 2   Child gets very upset if reminded of the event.

Source: Glenn N. Saxe, MD, and Michelle Bosquet, PhD, Center for Behavioral Science, Children's Hospital, Boston.

mother's side. On asking further, Ann learned that Tanya had been refusing food and sleeping only fitfully at night.

Children who are school-aged are at risk of several adverse outcomes well after the traumatic event. This was demonstrated in children after

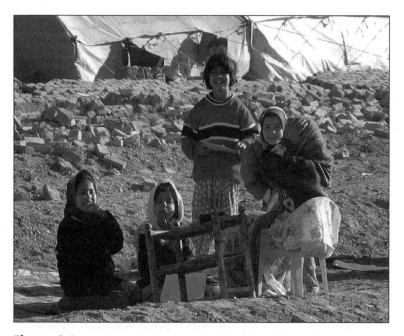

Figure 9.1 Children who survived the earthquake in Bam, Iran, 2003. *Source:* Courtesy of Jay Schnitzer, MD.

the 1996 Oklahoma City bombing. Many children knew someone who had been killed, and 20% remained symptomatic at a 2-year follow-up.[6] Although adults may minimize children's reactions and see them as transient, this is not true for those children most exposed to the event and its aftermath. Children from minority groups, such as Muslim children, may be harshly stigmatized by peers, such as after the attacks of 9/11. Under severe stress, including injuries, children may commonly regress with temporary loss of mastered skills such as speech, continence, academic skills, and interpersonal relatedness even up to early adolescence. The child approaching puberty may have greater difficulty in coping with maturational stresses when enduring a disaster and its effects, especially if his or her parents are unavailable.

Adolescents moving rapidly through puberty and into young adulthood experience shifts in cognition, emotional and physical maturation, and peer relations. Their abilities to endure stress vary widely, often depending on the degree of family, school, and community support they receive. The more vulnerable adolescents are those who were previously traumatized, have lost someone, are not achieving in school, or who suffer from a physical or mental illness. The vulnerable adolescent, especially if previously traumatized, is at risk for post-traumatic symptoms and depression, and he or she may engage in risky behaviors involving peers including sex, drugs, or aggression. If the adolescent thinks or feels that she may have contributed to an injury or a death, or if the adolescent is grieving, her guilty feelings may be intense and persistent. On the other hand, many adolescents cope adaptively by acting altruistically, protectively, or bravely, either spontaneously or with encouragement from adults. Adolescents and older children often feel more confidence and satisfaction, with greater self-esteem, in being able to help in a disaster response.

A key function for Ann will be her availability to teachers and other stressed members of the community who support children. Advising school or orphanage personnel or other community resources is an important component of her or any volunteer's role. She could discuss the basic principles, as outlined here, with community providers.

Families and Communities

Disasters often disrupt structures within families and the community, which otherwise nurture and protect children. As a result, the suffering of children may go on long after the original traumatic events, affecting lifelong psychological and neurobiological development. [2,7-9] In assessing the factors strengthening families' resiliency in the face of disaster, their extended family, occupational and educational supports, economic resources, religious affiliations, and ethnic and community ties are critical to consider.

Fathers in most parts of the world play a central role in the family but may be absent due to the need to work, secondary to being injured or killed, incarcerated, a refugee, or for other reasons. A father often must cope with the awareness that the disaster devastated his ability to work or provide basic needs for his family, often with great personal anguish. If he is present or available, it is essential to make efforts to include the father in the family assessment and to gain his cooperation with plans for intervention.

Psycho-education about the effects of disaster and trauma on the mental health of children and families is an important element of the outreach to all family members, including fathers. This may be difficult if men in the society consider health care for the family a duty of the women or if they distrust those providing disaster relief.

Credentialed child and family assistance centers, community agencies, and children's and family services provided through pediatric services, schools, community agencies, and religious organizations all provide essential community functions in the regular lives of children. It is therefore important to ensure that these entities are functioning or restored after a disaster, thereby maintaining as much normalcy and routine in the lives of affected children and adolescents as is possible under the circumstances. These agencies also contribute to the assessment of the impact of disasters and determine what the next steps should be for planning child and family mental health programming, as was seen following the 9/11 terrorist attacks and Hurricane Katrina.[1,10]

Conclusion

This chapter has briefly presented how to conduct a clinical assessment of a traumatized child, the effects of disasters at various developmental stages, and the importance of understanding the range of community resources upon which children and families depend. Ultimately, essential principles in assessing and intervening with disaster-affected children have been articulated in the three elements of psychological first aid for children and adolescents.[11] If in your work as a health care provider after a disaster you keep the following principles in mind, you will be practicing in a way that fundamentally provides for the mental well-being of the children and families you come into contact with:

Listen: Listen and pay attention to what children say and how they act.

Protect: Oversee children's day-to-day life in a way that provides them with an honest exposure to the situation without over-exposing them.

Connect: Reach out to friends, neighbors, teachers, and others in the community.

References

1. Saltzman WR, Layne CM, Steinberg AM, Arslanagic B, Pynoos RS. Developing a culturally and ecologically sound intervention program for youth exposed to war and terrorism. *Child Adolesc Psychiat Clin N Am.* 2003;12:2:319–342.

2. Weine S, Feetham S, Kulauzovic Y, et al. A family belief's framework for socially and culturally specific preventive interventions with refugee youths and families. *Am J Orthopsychiat.* 2006;76(1):1–9.

3. Stoddard F, Saxe G. Ten-year research review of physical injuries. *J Am Acad Child Adolesc Psychiatry.* 2001;40(10):1128–1145.

4. LaGreca AM, Silverman WK, Vernberg, EM, Roberts MC. *Helping Children Cope with Disasters and Terrorism.* Washington, DC: American Psychological Association; 2002.

5. Stoddard FJ, Menninger EW. Guidance for parents and other caretakers after disasters or terrorist attacks. In: Hall RCW, Ng AT, Norwood AE, Eds. *Disaster Psychiatry Handbook.* Available at: **http://www.psych.org/ Resources/DisasterPsychiatry/APADisasterPsychiatryResources/ DisasterPsychiatry Handbook.aspx**. Accessed March 18, 2009.

6. Gurwitch RH, Sitterle KA, Young BH, Pfefferbaum B. The aftermath of terrorism. In: LaGreca AM, et al., Eds. *Helping Children Cope with Disasters and Terrorism.* Washington, DC: American Psychological Association; 2002.

7. Cohen JA, Mannarino AP, Gibson LE, Cozza SJ, Brymer SJ, Murray L. Interventions for children and adolescents following disasters. In: Ritchie EC, Watson PJ, Friedman MJ, Eds. *Interventions Following Mass Violence and Disasters: Strategies for Mental Health Practice.* New York: The Guilford Press; 2006:227–256.

8. Farah MJ, Shera DM, Savage JH, Betancourt L, Giannetta JM, Brodsky NL, Malmud EK, Hurt H. Childhood poverty: specific associations with neurocognitive development. *Brain Res.* 2006;110:166–174.

9. Evans GW, Shamberg MA. Childhood poverty, chronic stress and adult working memory. Proceedings of the National Academy of Sciences. PNAS Early Edition. Available at: **http://www.pnas.org/content/106/16/6545**. Accessed April 10, 2009.

10. Saxe GN, Ellis BH, Kaplow J. *Collaborative Treatment of Traumatized Children and Teens: The Trauma Systems Therapy Approach.* New York: The Guilford Press; 2006.

11. Schreiber M, Gurwitch R. Listen, Protect, and Connect: Psychological First Aid for Children and Parents, 2006. Available at: **http://www.ready.gov/ kids/_downloads/PFA_SchoolCrisis.pdf**. Accessed March 15, 2008.

Medically Unexplained Physical Symptoms

10

Frederick J. Stoddard Jr., MD
Craig L. Katz, MD

You are a physician on duty in your urban emergency department 1 week after the first cases of inhalational anthrax become known and confirmed as a likely terrorist incident. Anna comes to triage asking for "Cipro" for anthrax exposure. She is a 37-year-old freelance writer and reports no significant past medical history. The triage nurse notes that she is afebrile, has stable vital signs, and appears mildly anxious. Given the apparent non-acuity of her presentation, she is asked to wait in the waiting room until a physician becomes available.

About an hour into her wait, Anna comes running up to the triage nurse, now complaining of shortness of breath and chest pain. She looks very anxious, sweaty, a little disheveled, and appears mildly short of breath. Her vital signs remain stable except for a respiratory rate that is now 20 instead of 12. Anna gets loud and yells, "If I do not get help, I will leave right now. I do not care if I spread this around the city." When attempts by the nurse to reassure the patient that someone will be with her soon lead her to become even louder, Anna is ushered into

- Medically unexplained physical symptoms (MUPS) refers to the clinical presentation many patients display after a disaster; these patients have no evidence of toxic exposure nor physical explanations for their symptoms.

- A four-tiered approach can be taken to identifying patients with serious medical conditions while progressively isolating those conditions that are probably due to MUPS.

- Clinical approaches to patients with MUPS include taking their complaints seriously while avoiding excessive testing and work-up.

the ED's sub-acute treatment area and assigned to you as her physician.

Upon interviewing Anna, you learn that she has had sweats, shortness of breath, and chest pain on and off since arriving back in the city from a 3-week vacation 2 nights ago. She said she "knows" it is anthrax. Upon further questioning, Anna indicated that she had never been in the telecommunications building though it is the site of the primary exposure nor has she received suspicious mail. She was also out of town at the time of the apparent exposures. You conclude that she is not likely to have been exposed and her subsequent unremarkable physical examination confirms this. You conclude that she does not need antibiotic prophylaxis.

Overview

Medically unexplained physical symptoms (MUPS) refer to the clinical presentation of many patients, like Anna, who after a disaster or terrorist attack, have no evidence of toxic exposure and no physical explanation for their symptoms. MUPS can strike people of all ages. The result is potentially to overwhelm primary care clinicians with people who fear that they have been contaminated or injured, when in fact their symptoms are psychosomatic in origin. This phenomenon is especially important to emergency services since they will usually be on the front lines of receiving casualties, whether physical or, as in MUPS, psychological.

If, as occurred after the 1995 sarin nerve agent attack in the Tokyo subway, hundreds or thousands of people seek emergency services, the capacity of those services is quickly overwhelmed, and the most severely injured may not be able to be served. In the Tokyo attack, the ratio of those with non-significant symptoms to those who died was about 500:1.[1] After a radiation accident in Brazil in 1987, the ratio of people with health anxieties to casualties was about 1700:1. As a result, the term "surge capacity" has evolved to describe the ability of emergency services to deal with a surge in mass casualties, which may include psychosomatic presentations. These go by various names such as medically unexplained symptoms (MUS), idiopathic physical symptoms (IPS), mass idiopathic physical symptoms, mass sociogenic illness, but MUPS is used here because it does not attribute to causality.[2,3] Although most people respond with compassion, offer mutual aid, and seek to reconnect with loved ones after disasters, a significant minority will be very distressed and may urgently seek medical help from you.

Potential Magnitude of the Problem

The idiopathic physical symptoms seen after supposed toxic exposure include dizziness, faintness, shortness of breath, nausea, palpitations, abdominal distress, and others.[4] These symptoms may spread rapidly through a population after a putative exposure. Mass idiopathic illness has been described as a result of an actual or rumored event of release of toxic waste, gas, water or food contamination, a suspicious odor, an infectious agent, or radiation. The 2001 anthrax scare set off a wave of symptoms in individuals who had no exposure.[5] Formerly called by the pejorative term "mass hysteria" such symptoms have been witnessed to spread rapidly in association with unexplained odors in settings such as schools. Fears of infection in hospitals during the SARS epidemic contributed to unexplained medical symptoms and to ethical dilemmas in provision of care to patients with SARS similar to such dilemmas in prior epidemics.[6] Due to overlapping symptoms, it can be difficult to distinguish MUPS from the symptoms of infection (e.g., from an epidemic or a bioterrorist contamination). Training in the ways that infectious disease, psychiatric disorders, and behavioral contagion present can help you to properly triage and manage these issues.[7]

The problems may be broader than medically unexplained symptoms, including the full range of types of distress, acute anxiety, and new and recurrent psychiatric problems and disorders, including increased substance use. In countries with centralized health care systems, resources can be shifted to provide personnel trained with needed mental health skills, but in the United States there are not efficient ways to "rectify the shortage of clinicians with trauma and grief experience."[8]

Systematic Approaches to the Problem

Careful planning needs to address problems of damage to the health care infrastructure, such as occurred after Hurricane Katrina and problems of rural populations, such as those after the 2004 tsunami in Asia, where health care facilities may be unavailable. Weisler et al have described the destruction of health and mental health care facilities, loss of patient records, problems with traveling to functioning health care facilities, and depletion of the physician workforce after Hurricane Katrina.[9] Yet even fully functioning health care systems could be derailed by people presenting with MUPS.

In seeking to prepare for the risk of MUPS overwhelming whatever health care infrastructure may be available, a large conference on MUPS was sponsored by the Centers for Disease Control and other agencies of the Department of Health and Human Services, Georgetown University, and other groups. From this conference, Engel et al proposed a progressive four-tier clinical intervention model for a health care system (Table 10.1) or an ad hoc screening facility to respond "to surging demands for triage and management in the event of mass idiopathic illness and overwhelming health anxiety."[4]

Level I

Level I is distance "tele-triage," allowing you "initial remote contact with a prospective patient by telephone, Internet, or other methods." You might provide instruction, education, and reassurance, enabling some patients to "shelter at home."[10]

Level II

Level II is when your patient undergoes a brief medical assessment for indicators of disease such as "inability to walk, signs of physical trauma, a sick or 'toxic' appearance, acute respiratory distress, and one or more

Table 10.1   Four-Tier MUPS Intervention Model

Level I: Distance tele-triage.

Level II: Brief medical assessment for indicators of disease.

Level III: Standardized review of systems, including a count of physical symptoms which is combined with standardized health anxiety ratings to identify MUPS symptoms.

Level IV: This depends on the nature of the event. Most patients would go home to await medical follow-up, which would emphasize continuity with a nurse or non-MD care manager, and watchful waiting with scheduled visits, self-care instruction, and the provision of health information.

unstable vital signs."[10] You would provide medical or surgical care to those who are most ill, while moving others to a medical holding area for the next level of assessment.

Level III

At Level III you obtain a standardized review of systems, including a count of physical symptoms. The count is combined with standardized health anxiety ratings assessed either by self-ratings or with an assistant using standard assessment protocols. The physical symptom count is combined with the health anxiety rating to identify MUPS symptoms. Your patients with idiopathic physical symptoms and health anxiety move to the next level.

Level IV

The location of Level IV care would depend on the nature of the event, but most patients would go home to await medical follow-up, whether with you or other providers in the community. Follow-up would emphasize "continuity with a nurse or non-physician care manager and watchful waiting consisting of scheduled visits, self-care instruction, and the provision of health information."[10] Brief semi-structured psychiatric self-assessment screening tools, adaptable to the Internet, could be used to identify treatable post-traumatic disorders.

Clinical Approaches to the Problem

Here are some ways to explain medical findings to patients you have concluded have MUPS:[10]

1. Express empathy for the patient's suffering and worry.
2. Inform the patient of the good news—there is no serious disease or injury.
3. Do not say there is nothing wrong.
4. Examine the patient's reaction to this news, and elicit the patient's explanation for his or her symptoms.
5. Correct misunderstandings about the patient's body and its function.
6. Explain in simple terms how anxiety may be related to experiencing bodily sensations; avoid psychiatric terminology.

7. Avoid arguing with your patients.
8. Above all, convey to your patient that you recognize his or her symptoms as a real and genuine reaction to a traumatic experience.

Thereafter, you can manage MUPS in some of the following ways:

1. Have one designated clinician assigned to the patient.
2. Focus on patient function rather than symptoms.
3. Explore psychosocial issues.
4. Prescribe benign treatments (leisure activities).
5. Offer close follow-up.

On the other hand, you should *not* manage MUPS in any of the following ways:

1. By telling your patients "it's all in your head"
2. Pursuing excessive invasive testing or procedures
3. Referring to specialists
4. Focusing on symptoms

References

1. Kawana N. Psycho-physiological effects of the terrorist sarin attack on the Tokyo subway system. *Military Medicine.* 2001;166(2):23–26.

2. Boss LP. Epidemic hysteria: a review of the published literature. *Epidemiol Rev.* 1997;19(2):233–243.

3. Mawson AR. Understanding mass panic and other collective responses to threat and disaster. *Psychiatry.* 2005;68(2):95–110.

4. Engel CC, Locke S, Reissman DB, et al. Terrorism, trauma, and mass casualty triage: how might we solve the latest mind-body problem. *Biosecurity Bioterrorism: Biodefense Strategy Practice Science.* 2007;5(2):1–9.

5. Bartholomew RE, Wessely S. Protean nature of mass sociogenic illness: from possessed nuns to chemical and biological terrorism fears. *Br J Psychiatry.* 2002;180:300–306.

6. Nickell LA, Crighton EJ, Tracy CS, et al. Psychosocial effects of SARS on hospital staff: survey of a large tertiary care institution. *CMAJ.* 2004;170:793–798.

7. Rundell JR, Christopher GW. Differentiating manifestations of infection from psychiatric disorders and fears of having been exposed to bioterrorism. In: Ursano RJ, Norwood AE, Fullerton CS, Eds. *Bioterrorism: Psychological*

and Public Health Interventions. Cambridge: Cambridge University Press; 2004;88–108.

8. Marshall RD. Learning from 9/11: implications for disaster research and public health. In: Neria Y, Gross R, Marshall R, Eds. *9/11: Mental Health in the Wake of Terrorist Attacks.* Cambridge: Cambridge University Press; 2006;422.

9. Weisler RH, Barbee JG, Townsend MH. Mental health and recovery in the Gulf Coast after Hurricanes Katrina and Rita. *JAMA.* 2006;296:585–588.

10. New York City Department of Health and Mental Hygiene in consultation with Disaster Psychiatry Outreach. *Mental Health Consequences of Bioterrorism: A Disaster Preparedness Course for Hospital Emergency Department Staff.* New York: NYC Department of Health and Mental Hygiene; 2004.

Difficult Encounters

Anthony T. Ng, MD

Mr. D is a single 35-year-old businessman with non-insulin dependent diabetes mellitus. Since a flood devastated his community, Mr. D has been staying at a Red Cross shelter. Previously fastidious in how he managed his diabetes, he has been ignoring his diet and blood sugar. He had been complaining of various pains and GI-related issues to the shelter nurse who referred him to you, the primary care clinician, after he was found to have hyperglycemia by finger stick. You become frustrated at Mr. D's continued failure to follow his diabetic regimen despite the availability of a proper diet and medications at the shelter. After verbalizing your disappointment to Mr. D, he replied, "I know, I know. I must be such a burden on you." You are increasingly annoyed with Mr. D's frequent visits to see you, as well as his numerous phone calls that seem to lead to little change. You are starting to feel Mr. D is taking up too much of your time. You are also stressed by having so many new patients to deal with while at the same time having to deal with flood damages to your own house.

- The chaos and stress of disasters can lead to extreme behaviors and emotions in otherwise "normal" patients.

- Clinicians may experience an usually large number of difficult encounters with their patients during times of disaster.

- There are at least four subtypes of difficult patient situations that may arise in a disaster, even in people who were not previously prone to such difficulties.

- An important first step for clinicians is to recognize and appreciate their own reactions to better help mitigate or resolve difficult patient encounters.

Overview

In our daily clinical work across the medical specialties, "difficult encounters" with patients are inevitable. Such situations may include patients who repeatedly need the attention of their clinicians, while refusing to adhere to medical advice or take the prescriptions given, as we see in the example of Mr. D. There may be others who take their frustrations out on their clinicians, including demeaning their recommendations or professionalism or being overtly rude and angry, possibly to the point of threatening legal action and even bodily harm. These difficult encounters may challenge your ability to provide good clinical care, all the while exacting a personal toll on you.

The likelihood of a clinician experiencing difficult encounters may be greater in the aftermath of a community-wide disaster or mass trauma. The post-disaster environment is often chaotic and fluid. The needs of individuals and communities may be many and in flux. Health care and other community resources may be scarce, disrupted, or even destroyed. Taken together, this can precipitate uncommon neediness and greater demands placed upon you by your patients. With a greater awareness of such potential situations, you can take steps to mitigate the impacts of such patient encounters on both your patients and yourself in the already taxing post-disaster period.

Types of Difficult Encounters

Groves has famously written of four types of difficult patient encounters that commonly arise in clinical work: the dependent clinger, entitled demander, manipulative help rejecter, and the self-destructive denier (Box 11.1).[1] With the dependent clingers, patients may be superficially pleasant and nice but present frequent and insatiable demands, possibly leading the clinician to try to avoid them. The entitled demander may be excessively needy all the while intimidating and de-valuing you. The manipulative help rejecter has bottomless needs that resist all of your efforts, even worsening the more you try to meet her needs. Lastly, the self-destructive denier involves a patient who engages in self-destructive behavior, such as persistent eating of excessive sweets despite uncontrollable hyperglycemia.

Box 11.1   The Four Difficult Patient Encounters

Dependent Clinger

Entitled Demander

Manipulative Help Rejecter

Self-destructive Denier

Source: Groves JE. Taking care of the hateful patient. *NEJM.* 1978; 298:883–887.

Comparable but likely more intense patient situations can arise out of the pressure of the post-disaster environment, even in patients who usually do not pose difficulties. In fact, whereas these four types of encounters were developed to characterize exchanges that occur in the health care setting, they may well be generalized to a broad range of behaviors that occur amid the de-stabilizing effects of a disaster. In the case of the dependent clinger, a patient who has experienced significant losses requires increased attention from you. This may be manifested in greater somatic concerns or frequency of contacts with you. It probably emanates from a less than conscious need to feel noticed and connected despite the painful isolation of trauma and grief.

The entitled demander takes the attitude that he has suffered losses in the disaster and had so many bad things happen that he deserves to be treated better. Entitled demanders take the attitude that the doctor must do everything to help him. Such help may extend beyond medical assistance, for example. The patient may want the primary care clinician to help with basic or social service needs, which, however desirable, may strain your ability to address the range of more direct health issues you are encountering. In all likelihood you are treating many people, including survivors as well as responders and are doing all you can to keep up. Even if you deem these non-medical issues relevant to a patient's well-being and have the time to help, you may still find it challenging to help due to the demanding tone of the entitled demander. As an enduring symbol of compassion and commitment, you, the physician, may be subject to a deluge of finger-jabbing demands. People can "regress" readily after a disaster, becoming child-like in their impatience and neediness. They are seemingly trying to become the center of your universe at a time when they otherwise feel lost in the universe as they once knew it.

During a flu outbreak for example, people who have taken on the role of the manipulative help rejecter could have health concerns that persist despite your best efforts. Nothing you do seems to allay their anxiety and adequately convey your conviction that they have no clinical evidence of infection. They remain convinced of having been exposed and insist that their symptoms are atypical and presage death. It is as though they feel they need to be sick in order to have any importance and get noticed. See Chapter 10 for more information on medically unexplained symptoms.

The self-destructive denier in the disaster setting can continue to engage in behavior that you feel is risky. For example, a responder with severe asthma and on steroids prior to a disaster continues to work long hours in the recovery environment where there are known asbestos and allergen exposures. They even flaunt the fact that they refuse to wear their OSHA recommended respiratory mask. Feeling uncommonly vulnerable amid all of the death and destruction, self-destructive deniers counter these feelings by acting as though they are invulnerable.

Importantly, people who are adherent and amiable patients under normal circumstances can suddenly be fueling any of these four types of encounters, if not others, during a disaster. Additionally, patients who have untreated psychiatric conditions such as clinical depression or PTSD may be needy, clingy, or even hostile. These symptoms would be compounded if they were drinking alcohol to help them cope. Pre-existing *DSM-IV* Axis II personality disorders (PD) or dysfunctional personality traits can also lead to such behavior. Individuals may behave more emotionally and chaotically in an already chaotic environment due to pre-existing disturbances in cognitive processing or affective stability and impulse control in individuals with PD. They may be seen as demanding, unreasonable, and have shifting priorities in dealing with their post-disaster needs (see Box 11.2).

Management of "Difficult" Encounters

Strategies for dealing with these difficult encounters are available. Before deciding what to do though, you should take a step back to think

Box 11.2 Post-Disaster Issues That May Affect Individuals With Personality Disorders

---

Direct injuries

Death or injuries to family, friends, and others to whom the individual seems close

Loss or disruption of familiar social support

Displacement and evacuation

Job loss

Financial loss

Chaos of disaster response, such as obtaining benefits, housing, etc.

Inconsistent information about the disaster

Pre-existing medical or psychiatric conditions

Substance abuse

Paranoia about causes of disaster (e.g., who is responsible, why it happened)

---

about how the involved patient(s) are making *you* feel.[2,3] These encounters, compounded by the global stresses of disaster work, may evoke negative feelings in you, such as anger, frustration, and feelings of helplessness. Unless identified and acknowledged, these feelings can lead you to avoid these individuals, to minimize their needs, or to respond unprofessionally and antagonistically. Unnoticed, they can even cloud the clarity of your decision making on their behalf.

The key for most providers is to be as supportive as possible. This can include setting limits on their behavior or even discussing how they treat you. Others will benefit from your help in prioritizing their needs. The positive and negative consequences of their actions and decisions can be highlighted so as to decrease and manage their impulsivity. Some individuals may benefit from frequent, regular, and brief follow-up, thereby offering them your attention and some structure amid the disruptions of the disaster environment.

More specifically, for the encounters with the dependent clinger, your interventions should focus on setting limits. Once this behavior emerges, such patients should be informed as soon as possible that you have limits not only in knowledge and skills but also in time and energy. Realistic expectations of the role of the clinician should be made clear and non-defensively reiterated to the patient.

With working clinically with entitled demanders, you can agree that they deserve the best. To strive toward that goal, patients should be encouraged not to fight or even threaten you. The patient's sense of entitlement should be channeled into an integrated regimen. For example, "I agree with your need to get the best as you or anyone deserves, but I need your help. I need your help in getting this care. Let's try to channel this anger and energy away from the very people who are trying to help you get that care."

For the manipulative help rejecter, the patient's pessimism toward cure should be acknowledged, but the clinician should also reinforce to the patient that she will not be abandoned and that perhaps brief, regular follow-up can be in place to "monitor" the patient's care. For the self-destructive denier, what a clinician can actually do may be limited. First and foremost it is important to recognize the clinician's own limits in how much he can realistically help the patient. Be mindful of so-called rescue behavior, whereby you try to save the patient from herself. This is especially so in the post-disaster environment when the needs of one individual must be balanced against the greater need of the community that has also been traumatized. The clinician needs to appreciate his limits and what is realistic in terms of the care that can be provided. Lastly, for the more severe self-destructive type of patients, formal psychiatric consultations, including hospital confinement, may be necessary.

Where relevant, addressing Axis I major clinical disorders and Axis II personality disorders can help mitigate and minimize the impact of these encounters on both the patient and the clinician. To the extent that it is available, pharmacotherapy may be helpful.[4,5] For depression, antidepressants such as SSRIs may be used. Intense anxiety may also respond to SSRI treatment, with some adjunct use of benzodiazepines for severe anxiety. If the latter is used, it should be used for a short term; be cautious of the potential abuse nature of benzodiazepines. Mood stabilizers or second-generation antipsychotics (SGA) may be helpful for some with affective instability.

If you have access to mental health professionals, psychotherapies may be used for some patients with mild to moderate depression and some cognitive distortions, including those with PDs or persistently dysfunctional behavior.[6–8] These may be especially important if you do not have ready access to usual psychotropic medications. Potential psychotherapy approaches include supportive (focusing on crisis management); exploratory (focusing on their mind and longstanding ways of thinking or feeling that are unconsciously coloring their reaction to the situation); or cognitive-behavioral (addressing dysfunctional patterns in which they interpret the world, themselves, or others).

References

1. Groves JE. Taking care of the hateful patient. *NEJM*. 1978;298:883–887.

2. Rossberg JI, Karterud S, Pedersen G, et al. An empirical study of countertransference reactions toward patients with personality disorders. *Compr Psychiatry*. 2007;48:225–230.

3. Betan E, Heim AK, Zittel Conklin C, et al. Countertransference phenomena and personality pathology in clinical practice: an empirical investigation. *Am J Psychiatry*. 2005;162:890–898.

4. Gitlin MJ. Pharmacotherapy of personality disorders: conceptual framework and clinical strategies. *J Clin Psychpharmacol*. 1993;13:343–353.

5. Hori A. Pharmacotherapy for personality disorders. *Psychiatry Clin Neurosci*. 1998;52:13–19.

6. Stone MH. Clinical guidelines for psychotherapy for patients with borderline personality disorder. *Psych Clin N Am*. 2000;23:193–210.

7. Verheul R, Herbrink M. The efficacy of various modalities of psychotherapy for personality disorders: a systemic review of the evidence and clinical recommendations. *Int Rev Psychiatr*. 2007;19:25–38.

8. Winston A, Laikin M, Pollack J, et al. Short-term psychotherapy of personality disorders. *Am J Psychiatry*. 1994;151:190–194.

Special Populations in Disaster: The Impact of Gender, Culture, Age, and Severe and Persistent Mental Illness

Kristina Jones, MD

Following a massive tornado that devastated a medium-size town, Angela, a 29-year-old woman with a prior history of bipolar disorder, was asked by her employer to work at a disaster site in a food service tent near the staging area for responders. She was encouraged to stay at a hotel that was being used as a sleeping facility for workers. During the night, an unknown worker or member of the public forced his way into the hotel room and attempted to rape her. Angela fended him off and spent the remainder of the night watching the cranes clear the rubble. She did not tell anyone what had happened to her. She continued working under tremendous anxiety and fear but was worried that if she asked to leave, her employer would think she was a "wimp," and merely being difficult. Angela remained at the site for 5 days, unable to sleep, and sought shelter in the church nearby for part of the following nights. She reported that during the sleep deprivation and without her medication, she became manic, with irritable mood, grandiosity, and pressured speech, behavior that friends interpreted as demonstrating tremendous courage and heroism. On

- Certain groups within the community may suffer unique psychological strains, and health care providers can advocate for them.

- A number of factors may place women at higher risk for psychiatric sequelae of disasters.

- Be aware of culture-specific interpretations and reactions to disaster.

- Some of the elderly may present with a combination of social, physical, and emotional needs.

- The chronically mentally ill may become lost to treatment and crucial support systems after a disaster.

referral by Gina, an NP working with Peter, Angela came to psychiatric attention 3 months later when her employer fired her for not being able to control her irritability. Lacking health insurance after losing her job, she presented to a federal program asking for medication assistance and was then referred to a mental health program for free medication and counseling by a social worker.

Introduction

Disaster affects the community as a whole, and although a catastrophic event can sometimes unify disparate groups, victims of the same disaster can have very different experiences of the event. Though disaster is often perceived to be a great leveler, the outcome is not the same for everyone.[1,2] Disaster will have different effects on special populations with relatively similar demographics. Examples include women, who have higher rates of depression and prior trauma; cultural groups with alternative philosophies of why disasters happen and how to care for themselves afterward; children and the elderly, who are at the vulnerable extremes of age; and people with severe and persistent mental illness, who often have fragile support networks and poor socioeconomic status; refugees and immigrants, and others who are poor and vulnerable. You are certain to encounter members of these special populations in the course of your disaster work, and such patients may present challenges for the medical clinician. This chapter will help to highlight mental health issues specific to women, cultural groups, the elderly, and those with severe and persistent mental illness (SPMI).

Gender

Women are at increased risk for disaster-related disorders. Research indicates that female gender is itself a risk factor.[3] Women have higher pre-existing rates of anxiety, depression, and trauma, including sexual trauma, and prior history is a risk factor during disaster or post-disaster. After the Chernobyl nuclear disaster, women had increased rates of anxiety at a rate of four-to-fivefold greater than men, and a threefold greater risk for any psychiatric disorder.[4] Having young children further

increased the risk for women. For women whose husbands are injured or killed in disasters, the burden of becoming the sole or primary financial caretaker in addition to providing childcare or care of elders is significant. Especially in disasters where war is a feature, women are often targeted for rape and physical violence or mutilation. Women are also more vulnerable when separated from usual cohabitation arrangements with men or when men are displaced. Poverty, whether chronic or new, is an added burden for women in many disaster situations.

Cultural Groups

Minority groups may draw different meanings from disaster than nonminorities. For example, some groups affected by disaster, such as some Latino communities, may possess a belief in Fatalism, a system that attributes the external environment with a causal power.[5] For example, "susto," or fright sickness, is a medical condition seen in some Latino patients. The patient attributes a wide range of physical symptoms to a frightening experience and names this constellation of symptoms after the "susto" or fright. In contrast, most non-Hispanic Western cultures possess a belief in instrumentalism, a system that considers the individual responsible for most events, or if not the event, then the self-determining actions needed to help oneself regain full independence after a disaster.

You can anticipate that working with cultures whose basic interpretation of disaster involves fatalism requires an adjustment to your own more instrumentalist style. You should also be aware of historical animosities and current conflicts that may exist between your culture and that of your patients. Care should also be taken not to over-diagnose psychosis or agitation in cultures where belief in malevolent forces may be common and where loud emotional displays of grief or distress may be the norm.

In your role as a medical provider, your advice is likely to carry great authority, and you should use this influence to encourage your patients to use existing assets within their culture rather than to impose Western styles of coping on the patient. The patient's community must be accessed to provide group support. The promotion of a strong sense of belonging is an effective means to guard against real and perceived isolation, and it is especially helpful for members of disenfranchised cultural

groups. In the aftermath of 9/11, for example, Catholic churches were instrumental in organizing support groups for Polish workers affected by their experience at Ground Zero. Such groups organized informal networking, provided free meals, and offered pastoral counseling, since many of the Polish workers needed to process the event in a religious context, and because they sought to gain reassurance and safety from leaders in whom they had confidence. In your role as a psychologically attuned health care provider, you can educate these leaders about different forms of distress so that they can refer community members to professional medical providers when necessary.

Cultural Groups—Impact Phase

The cultural considerations you will encounter can vary with the timing of the disaster. During the impact phase (initial hours to a few days), be aware that any culture may have a different help-seeking behavior, including avoiding medical or mental health care due to stigma. Physical presentations of anxiety and distress may be widespread. Fear of deportation or discovery of non-visa status may be common, and language barriers are significant. Prior exposure to trauma means that some patients will become acutely anxious or numb and may be too dazed or detached to mobilize their own resources. During interviewing, recognize that direct questions may be perceived as shaming or confrontational. Be empathetic and ask for guidance from the patient or family about cultural norms of presentation of symptoms and the patient's past response to trauma.

Cultural Groups—Acute Phase

In the acute phase that spans from days to weeks after a disaster, recognize that there may be problems when interviewing using translators who might have their own cultural bias and therefore may compound mental health stigma by minimizing the patient's distress and symptoms. Some cultures hold the view that victims should endure distress rather than seek help, or keep distress private or among family members, while others might view help-seeking as a sign of weakness. There may be an expectation that the medical professional will offer material support, such as bus fare, or food, in addition to, or in lieu of, medical or mental health care.

Cultural groups may expect direct advice or instruction and not readily understand a collaborative approach that offers choices and requires self-help. Follow-up is always problematic due to financial concerns. Give your patients written instructions for follow-up and time frames during which they must call for appointments. This is more instructive for patients than the expectation that they must determine when they need help again or assess the efficacy of their medication.

Elderly

Researchers are divided over whether elderly members of the community are at increased risk for adverse mental health outcomes from disaster or whether advanced age may in fact be protective.[6] On the one hand, risk factors do aggregate, and elderly members of African American, Latino, and Eastern European immigrant communities may be at higher risk. On the protective side, the elderly may be better prepared or inoculated against trauma, and their lifetime of experience may serve as a source of wisdom. In some cases, short-term memory impairment might protect against psychiatric illness, but it also might pose a problem in accessing social services such as home care. Physical frailty or lack of funds may prevent the elderly from standing in line for aid, and they may have difficulty finding transportation to aid centers. The frail elderly are also at increased risk for dehydration and malnourishment. Additionally, the elderly may fear placement in a nursing home if they seek disaster-related help, and they are frequently easy victims of crime or charity scams. Active outreach is necessary to provide care in these situations. In the United States, groups such as Americorps, the VA hospitals, and the Red Cross can be alerted to the needs of elderly in the community.

Elderly—Impact Phase

During the impact phase of a disaster, be alert for cognitive decompensation in elderly patients and for presentations of delirium in those who have not consumed food or water or who have suffered even small injuries. Medical work-up should be a key part of your mental health assessment of elderly patients. Also, often due to lack of access to a pharmacy, common in the elderly population is lack of attention to

daily, long-term cardiac or blood pressure medications. Be mindful of the potential for increased alcohol consumption in some elderly patients. Though for some, visual and hearing impairments may result in decreased awareness of disaster. Others with such impairments may grow fearful because they lack the ability to protect themselves from physical harm.

Elderly—Acute Phase

In the acute phase of disaster, consider referring your elderly patients to still-functioning community services, even though they may imagine that regaining their independence will not be difficult or they fear that accepting such assistance will lead to placement in a nursing home. The need for such referrals decreases if patients have robust support systems, whether in the guise of a spouse, children or grandchildren, or friends. Those with dementia may exhibit acute behavioral dyscontrol syndrome in the face of a relocation or acute bereavement.

Pre-Existing Severe and Persistent Mental Illness

Patients with documented psychiatric disability are often among the most disenfranchised members of the community. Some are homeless; many live in single room occupancies. Others are in volatile housing situations with relatives or in illegal housing without the protection of a lease. They also have histories of trauma, which is an additional risk factor for developing psychiatric symptoms during a disaster. The National Comorbidity Study noted that up to 30% to 40% of the severely mentally ill also have comorbid PTSD.[7] The chronically mentally ill may become even more disenfranchised after a disaster. Following Hurricane Katrina, for example, there were widespread reports of refusal to allow mentally ill patients into shelters.[8] You must be their advocate. See Table 12.1 for a summary of the issues and interventions related to these efforts.

Pre-Existing Severe and Persistent Mental Illness— Impact Phase

Although some experts feel that psychotic patients may be oblivious to the scale of disaster, be alert to the fact that relapse can be rapid in the

Table 12.1 Severely and Persistently Mentally Ill: Disaster Stressors and Interventions

Vulnerable Populations:

Homeless.
Mentally ill in SROs (single room occupancies).
Schizophrenic patients.
Schizophrenic patients unstably housed with relatives, friends, on streets.
Schizophrenic patients with co-morbid cocaine, alcohol, or substance abuse.
Severe bipolar patients out of psychiatric care.

Acute Phase

Non-compliance with medication.
Acute disorganization, over-stimulation, increasing paranoia.
Delusions, increasing irritability, anger, and assaultive behavior.
Relapse of substance abuse.

Interventions:

Voluntary or involuntary admission to psychiatric hospital.
Dispensing antipsychotic medication from ER.
Use of pharmaceutical samples if patient unable to access pharmacy or day care.
Detoxification.
Mobilization of community centers, church programs to decrease isolation and provide structured setting.

Post-Acute Phase

Worsening psychosis, development of mania with irritability, potential aggression.
Relapse on cocaine, alcohol, or other substances.
Ongoing noncompliance with medication.
Lack of access to day treatment programs.
De-stabilization of housing.

Interventions:

Voluntary or involuntary admission to psychiatric hospital.
Provision or dispensing of medication from ER or disaster services.
Referral to medical detoxification or 28-day substance abuse rehabilitation center.
Referral to community agencies for social support, re-housing, crisis intervention teams.
Re-referral to psychiatric day care centers when available.
Advocacy and case management for access to medical and psychiatric services.
Referral to social services for case management.

schizophrenic population. Delusional patients may believe that their anger and hatred caused the disaster or they may believe that the forces or people who have been low-level sources of paranoia rose up and attacked. Many SPMI patients stop their medication because they no longer have access to it or because they become acutely disorganized. SPMI patients experience insomnia like others affected by disaster, but they are often more severely affected by fatigue and may suffer extreme irritability.

Pre-Existing Severe and Persistent Mental Illness— Acute Phase

During the acute phase of a disaster, pre-existing conditions can worsen. For example, some patients with bipolar disorder are highly vulnerable to the emergence of manic symptoms (lack of sleep, irritability, grandiosity, pressured speech) during times of extreme stress. Be alert to interruptions of treatment. Day programs and mental health appointments are often the "glue" that keeps the person with severe bipolar disorder or schizophrenia organized in terms of daily living. Such services and treatment facilities may not be available after a disaster. Therefore, if you are treating such a patient, refer them to a drop-in center, crisis center, or church-run facility where personal contact, activities, distraction, food, and social and spiritual support can help the patient avoid isolation and can help mitigate feelings of helplessness and vulnerability.

Always ask patients with psychiatric histories whether they have altered their dosage or timing of medication. Some patients may have missed monthly neuroleptic injections or started to ration their medication. Always assess for a new onset or relapse of substance abuse on cocaine, marijuana, or alcohol.

Conclusion

Special populations are those who rely on medical and mental health providers for their health and well-being at times of non-crisis and non-disaster. In a disaster setting, patients with different cultural backgrounds may present an assessment challenge because of psychosomatic complaints or their belief that nothing can be done to improve their mental health. Women are at higher risk for psychiatric sequelae of disaster, particularly those of lower socioeconomic status or with pre-existing depression or anxiety. Elderly patients may present to the ER with confusion, and mental health needs can be easily addressed at that time. Those with severe and persistent mental illness will have continuing needs and will not bear the additional burdens of disaster as well as others without pre-existing conditions. Remaining alert to the needs of special populations is an effective means to prevent patient relapse and to protect the most vulnerable members of our community.

References

1. Herman D, Felton C, Susser E. Mental health needs in New York State following the September 11th attacks. *J Urban Health: Bull NY Acad Med.* 2002;79(3):322–331.

2. Norris FH, Perilla JL, Ibañez GE, Murphy AD. Sex differences in symptoms of post-traumatic stress: does culture play a role? *J Traumatic Stress.* 2001;14(1):7–28.

3. Norris F, Friedman M, Watson, P. 60,000 disaster victims speak: part II. summary and implications of the disaster mental health research. *Psychiatry.* 2002;65(3):240–260.

4. Bromet E, Parkinson D, Schulberg H, Dunn L, Gondek P. Mental health of residents near the Three Mile Island reactor: a comparative study of selected groups. *J Preventive Psychiatry.* 1982;1(3):225–276.

5. Disaster Psychiatry Outreach. *The Essentials of Disaster Psychiatry: A Training Course for Psychiatrists.* New Canaan, CT: Disaster Psychiatry Outreach; April, 2008. Available at: **http://www.disasterpsych.org**. Accessed February 7, 2009.

6. Norris F, Friedman M, Watson P, Byrne C, Diaz E, Kaniasty K. 60,000 disaster victims speak: part I. an empirical review of the empirical literature 1981–2001. *Psychiatry.* 2002;65(3):207–239.

7. Bromet E, Sonnega A, Kessler RC. Risk factors for *DSM-III-R* post-traumatic stress disorder: findings from the National Comorbidity Survey. *Am J Epidemiol.* 1998;147(4):353–361.

8. National Council on Disability. *The Needs of People with Psychiatric Disabilities During and After Hurricanes Katrina and Rita.* Position Paper and Recommendations. Washington, DC: National Council on Disability; 2006.

Bereavement and Disasters

Knight Aldrich, MD

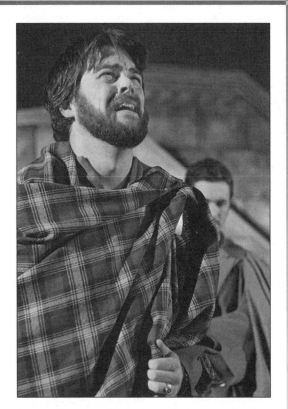

- The high mortality of disasters requires familiarity with all facets of bereavement.

- Attention to issues of bereavement should not be lost amid emergency care and triage.

- Acute grief reactions and prolonged grief reactions are the main concerns of the health care professional caring for bereaved survivors of disaster.

Source: Courtesy of Saint John Shakespeare Festival, www.saintjohnshakespeare.ca.

Ross brings the news to Macduff that Macbeth's minions have killed Macduff's wife and all of his children. Macduff at first says nothing, whereupon Malcolm urges him to communicate his feelings to his friends, saying, "Give sorrow words; the grief that does not speak whispers the o'er fraught heart and bids it break." Macduff at first cannot believe the tragedy that has befallen him. "My children, too?" he asks; then, "My wife, too?" and a little later, "All my pretty ones? . . . Did you say all?"[1]

Summarized from Act IV, Scene 3 of Shakespeare's *Macbeth*

Overview

Bereavement is the loss of someone or something held dear, whereas grief is the emotional accompaniment of bereavement. Mourning, sometimes called "grief work," involves actively participating in the socio-cultural process of coping with bereavement. Acute grief after losing loved ones in a disaster, such as Macduff experiences, may be truly unbearable, and the person may be held together only by the compassionate presence of another. The symptoms and signs of grief are both physiological and psychological and often resemble those of depression and anxiety. Yet symptoms vary widely from those easily recognizable as grief to somatoform pain or fatigue. Differentiating one from another may help in determining how you respond and provide treatment to a grieving person.

The Course of Grief

Most grieving people gradually come to grips with their losses without professional assistance. The usual course of grief starts with a brief period of being stunned or overwhelmed and progresses through months of yearning for the return of the deceased, often accompanied by denial, to a final acceptance of the loss, often with depression, and then to a period of restructuring the life of the survivor.[2]

In as many as 30% of the bereaved, however, this adaptation does not proceed smoothly and various complications of grief ensue. These complications usually include a prolongation of grief and the mourning process, a delay in getting the processes started, physical illness, or mental illnesses, such as major depression. As a health care professional in the disaster setting, you will encounter death and dying on a scale that is likely unfamiliar to you, and your future patients, as well as you, will benefit from anticipating the various needs that will arise around bereavement.

Help for the Bereaved Following Disaster

At a time of disaster you are likely to become involved in one or more of the following tasks involving bereaved persons:

Triage at an emergency department or similar site

Identification, diagnosis, care, and disposition of people with *acute grief reactions*

Identification, diagnosis, care, and disposition of patients with *complicated grief disorders*

After a disaster, triage screening is usually carried out in emergency settings so that first priority can be given to those for whom immediate care will make the difference between life and death. People with grief reactions are usually moved to a separate setting. Although sequestration may be necessary, it may have adverse consequences, three of which are listed below. These consequences usually can be avoided if you can anticipate them:

1. *Failure to care for relatives of patients who die while under emergency care.* Many next of kin are in need of counseling on site, not only for humanitarian reasons but also because caring for them can reduce their overt manifestations of grief that can lower morale in the emergency setting.

2. *Failure to care for people with symptoms of bereavement.* In the aura of surgical urgency that inevitably permeates emergency service areas, a sequestered group of grieving people may be forgotten and their needs overlooked. Even if physicians are in too short a supply, one or more members of the health care team, even if not part of the mental health staff, should be assigned to areas where grieving people are gathering or being gathered.

3. *Failure to provide grief counseling for patients under emergency medical care.* These injured patients may themselves be grieving for relatives or friends who have died in the disaster. Lindemann's pioneering work in the study of acute grief after the Coconut

Grove fire of 1942 was carried out with patients who were hospitalized with severe burns from that nightclub fire, their grieving relatives, and other grieving patients and relatives.[3]

Acute Grief

What will help most to facilitate grief work and to prevent the complications of grief is being an empathic listener. This includes avoiding trying prematurely to reassure or to stop the flow of emotion of the grieving person. You can also help the bereaved person to put feelings like guilt and shame into perspective.

Most of what is written here assumes that you and the bereaved share basic cultural views about bereavement. That is not always the case— even just talking to a stranger about one's grief can be inappropriate behavior in some cultures. Helping such patients to locate and talk with their spiritual advisors can help. These problems occur not only in foreign countries but also in settings like New York after the 9/11 terrorist attacks or New Orleans after Hurricane Katrina.

After a disaster, however, a person's trusted confidants may not be available, and responders may be the only ones to help the bereaved get started on their grief work. The passage from Shakespeare at the beginning of the chapter provides a dramatic example of acute grief that is as valid today as it was 400 years ago. In this brief excerpt, Macduff demonstrates the kind of initial inability to cope with overwhelming loss often seen in the relatives of disaster victims. Most bereaved people yearn for the return of the deceased and attempt unconsciously to deny the finality of the loss. This stage, as Joan Didion says in *The Year of Magical Thinking*, includes such evidence of denial as not throwing away her dead husband's old shoes because "he might need them when he comes back."[4] Denial performs a protective function here—it keeps the bereaved person from being overwhelmed and does not need to be refuted unless it is causing problems (as in the later example of prolonged grief).

The bereaved also express feelings of guilt and shame, sometimes deserved, but more often exaggerated or unrealistic. Macduff realistically if painfully goes on to speak of the guilt he feels for having left his family unguarded. "Sinful Macduff!," he says, "They were all struck for thee . . .

not for their own demerits but for mine fell slaughter on their souls."[1] As with denial, there is seldom a need to counter exaggerated or even unjustified guilt with more than an expression of mild perplexity—of not quite understanding why the bereaved is feeling guilt or shame

Grief is not an illness but a normal response to a life event. It is an event, however, that significantly increases the grieving person's vulnerability to the series of illnesses called "complicated grief," and that, especially early in its course, usually benefits from counseling. In any given disaster, there may not be enough professionals, including those providing mental health services and pastoral care, who can be assigned the role of providing grief counseling. Attending to grief in the course of medical care, therefore, may be an efficient way for you to participate as de facto "grief counselors."

It is important that community leaders—like Macduff—are not left out. Counseling may be necessary to permit them to carry out their leadership functions and to maintain morale. Since high morale that depends on confidence in leadership is a major determinant of effective coping in crises of any kind, you are helping the morale of the community at large when you help their leaders cope with their own grief. If you are unable to counsel them, be sure someone is identified and skilled enough who can.

Finally, different cultures have different ways of paying respect to the dead. In most cases, however, the observances also facilitate the survivors' grief work. So even though funeral and memorial ceremonies may take valuable time from necessary disaster recovery activities, remember that they contribute to the early management of bereavement as well as to community morale.

Prolonged Grief[5,6]

An example of a case of prolonged grief with continuing denial is England's Queen Victoria. Victoria, who became queen in 1837 at the age of 18, married Prince Albert 3 years later and became highly dependent on him. In her administrative duties he regularly gave her sound advice that was tailored to the times. After he died, she never stopped grieving. Along with having his bath drawn and pajamas laid out every night for the next 20 years, she continued to look to him for advice. All she could find was the advice he had given her before he died and that became more and more outdated as the years went by. As a result she was more and more often bypassed. Fortunately there were no serious disasters or other crises during this period.[5]

Such prolonged grief can be very complicated to manage and, if you were the physician to Queen Victoria or someone like her, you should strongly consider referral to a mental health professional. However, motivating her to do so would require great sensitivity.

Prolonged Grief—Possible Major Depression

Complicated grief may be difficult to diagnose, as in the case of Malcolm, the heir apparent to the Scottish throne whose father Macbeth was murdered. The episode also comes from Act IV, Scene 3 of *Macbeth*. Macduff has expected Malcolm to be eager to join his rebellion against Macbeth, but instead Malcolm hangs back, suspecting that Macduff will betray him to Macbeth—that he will "offer up a weak, poor, innocent lamb to appease an angry god." Malcolm's suspicion is accompanied by a detailed description of himself as such an evil character in every conceivable way that when people know him as he really is, "black Macbeth will seem as pure as snow."[1]

Macduff is surprised, offended, and deeply disappointed by Malcolm's response. He takes Malcolm literally and concludes that the young prince's character rules him out as a king. This is a crucial decision, and Macduff is about to abandon the whole rebellion when Malcolm, suddenly and miraculously won over by Macduff's sincerity, abandons his suspicions and evil intentions and becomes ready to join the rebellion—perhaps a sign of coping that psychotic people can manifest under extreme stress. Understandably, Macduff is confused, as are we. He hesitates, and when Malcolm asks him why, Macduff says, "Such welcome and unwelcome things at once, 'tis hard to reconcile."[1]

Shakespeare has a tendency to extricate his characters from complex situations through miracles that are indeed often "hard to reconcile." Malcolm's behavior, however, has suggested an illness, major depression, that is a frequent complication of grief, an illness to which Malcolm has become more vulnerable by leaving his entire support system immediately after the murder of his father in order to escape the same fate. At this point, Malcolm requires a formal mental health assessment.

Were you to encounter him in your practice, whether in times of disaster or otherwise, you would ask a number of questions:

1. Are Malcolm's suspicions paranoid and is his self-vilification delusional?
2. Is Malcolm mentally ill or is he a lonely adolescent, unsure if he has any friends and afraid of the responsibilities he is being asked to undertake?
3. If the former, is he suicidal? And if the latter, will he be able, with support, to meet the challenges of kingship? In other words, what is Malcolm's prognosis?

If today's Malcolm does have a major depression that includes psychotic thinking, he would probably require hospitalization and medication, neither of which may be available in the wake of a disaster. Otherwise, he may not be fit to assume his leadership role. You may find it necessary to transfer such patients to mental health facilities away from the disaster site for appropriate care if this kind of disposition is possible. Hospital facilities as well as supplies of medication, prescription records, doctors to write prescriptions, pharmacists to fill them, and communications to connect them with each other may all be missing after disasters. In this case, you may need to rely on whatever local supports are available to help keep the patient safe. The most likely response to help the person you are seeing in sorrow as a result of losing loved ones in a disaster comes from those words by Shakespeare, from Malcolm to Macduff: *"Give sorrow words; the grief that does not speak. Whispers the o'er fraught heart and bid its break."*[1]

References

1. Shakespeare W. *The Riverside Shakespeare.* Boston: Houghton Mifflin Company; 1974: 1332–1334.
2. Parkes CM, Ed. *Coping With Loss.* London: BMJ Books; 1998.
3. Lindemann E. The symptomatology and management of acute grief. *Am J Psychiatry.* 1944;101:141–147.
4. Didion J. *The Year of Magical Thinking.* New York: Random House; 2005.
5. Prigerson HG, Maciejewski PK. Grief and acceptance as opposite sides of the same coin: setting a research agenda to study peaceful acceptance of loss. *Br J Psychiatry.* 2008;193:435–437.

6. Prigerson HG, Vanderwerker LC, Maciejewski PK. Prolonged grief disorder: a case for inclusion in DSM-V. In: Stroebe M, Hansson R, Schut H, Stroebe W, Eds. *Handbook of Bereavement Research and Practice: 21st Century Perspectives.* Washington, DC: American Psychological Association Press; 2008.

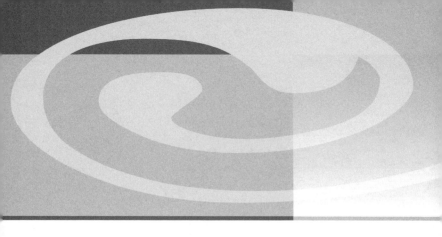

3

Intervention

Section Editor: Frederick J. Stoddard, Jr., MD

Psychological First Aid

Anthony T. Ng, MD
Edward M. Kantor, MD

Ms. J came to see her primary care physician, Dr. Jones, after recently witnessing her apartment building collapse, killing several members of her family. Ms. J, who has no prior psychiatric history, was noted by Dr. Jones to be anxious. Dr. Jones sat with Ms. J and listened to her concerns, which included worries about how to care for remaining members of her family as well as financial concerns stemming from the increased demands she now experienced. Dr. Jones talked with Ms. J about her temporary residence and where she may get financial assistance. She asked one of her clinic's social workers to see Ms. J. She also reminded Ms. J of her significant social supports including her large extended family, friends, and her church, and she was encouraged to use those supports.

- Psychological first aid (PFA) is delivery of pragmatic-oriented interventions in the early phases of disaster.

- PFA does not presume an individual to have psychiatric pathology from disaster.

- PFA encourages you to establish a human connection in a non-intrusive, compassionate manner.

- PFA facilitates the maintenance of individual functional capacities after disasters.

- PFA focuses on safety, social support, and efficacy (e.g., constructive activities, prioritizing needs).

Overview

Finding the right interventions to support the mental and psychosocial well-being of those exposed to disaster and mass trauma is a constantly evolving process. Not everyone develops mental illness following a disaster. In fact, most people do not. As noted in earlier chapters, the range and intensity of emotional reactions and the subsequent need for behavioral health supports are quite widespread. Although there are more than enough disasters, the research on what works and what doesn't—or what might even be harmful—has significantly lagged behind. While several modalities, such as cognitive behavioral therapy and desensitization training, have been found to benefit survivors of trauma, their applications in disaster and mass casualty incidents remain inconsistent. Due to the chaotic and fluid nature of such mass trauma events, studies evaluating the effectiveness of interventions remain difficult to implement. However, through an appreciation and understanding of risk and recovery factors, stress and traumatic stress theory, and expert consensus recommendations, an evidence-informed approach following the premises of psychological first aid (PFA) has been identified and endorsed by several reputable groups and findings. [1-4]

Background

Historically, PFA has been thought of as an approach for lay counselors and paraprofessionals early after exposure, much like regular first aid is in cases of physical trauma—stop the bleeding, splint the fracture, and refer those in need of more definitive treatment to emergency rooms or their own physicians. Rather than limiting PFA to paraprofessionals, it may make more sense to define its appropriateness by setting and context regardless of whether you are a nurse, an emergency medical technician, a primary care physician, or a psychiatrist. PFA could involve the concomitant use of psychopharmacology to achieve its goals but goes well beyond this option. More information on psychopharmacology in the aftermath of disasters is addressed in Chapter 18 later in this section.

PFA is a modular approach that entails pragmatic interventions during the immediate impact phase (initial days to weeks) to individuals experiencing acute reactions to the stress of a disaster (e.g., physical, psychological, cognitive, and spiritual). Signs of distress may include being disoriented, confused, feeling panicky, extremely withdrawn, apathetic or "shut down," as well as being extremely irritable, angry, or showing excessive worries. PFA specifically does not assume that all survivors will develop diagnosable psychopathology but is made available to those at risk of significant distress. PFA responds to presenting symptoms and circumstances with easily applied interpersonal and psychosocial interventions. PFA helps to facilitate the maintenance of functioning capacity of individuals after a disaster. It is intended to promote adaptive coping and to enhance problem solving both in the short and long term. This can help individuals after disasters deal with many post-disaster issues, such as basic needs for shelter, food, and water. PFA can facilitate individuals seeking post-disaster services from the various human services agencies. PFA includes assessment of needs and concerns of survivors, providing practical assistance, assisting individuals with reconnection to social supports, providing information to survivors on distress reactions and coping, and, last, assisting survivors with linkages to collaborative services.

The principles and techniques of PFA have been demonstrated to be appropriate from early childhood to the elderly, encompassing all developmental levels across the life span as well as being culturally informed and adaptable. PFA has been identified as an effective tool for response personnel, including primary care clinicians, to utilize in the acute aftermath of disaster.[5] Recognizing that there are many agencies and courses utilizing PFA concepts, for the purpose of this book, the *PFA Field Guide* created for the Medical Reserve Corps (MRC), by the National Child Traumatic Stress Network (NCTSN) and the National Center for Post-Traumatic Stress Disorder (NCPTSD), is highlighted along with additional descriptions from consensus between the American Red Cross, the Centers for Disease Control and Prevention, and the American Psychoanalytic Association.[6,7] The description of PFA here and in Boxes 14.1 and 14.2 is an introduction and does not substitute for a PFA course with practical skills sessions and instructor guidance. Readers are strongly encouraged to obtain the full PFA training through their local MRC, the American Red Cross, or another reputable training organization. There is a free, online introduction to PFA that is true to the concepts presented here and provides an excellent overview of the philosophy, concepts, and techniques (**http://pfa.naccho.org/pfa/pfa_ start.html**).[8] Again, it is not a substitute for practical exercises and supervised experience.

Fetter summarized PFA as focusing on safety, social support, and efficacy.[7] In terms of safety, survivors' basic needs and physical concerns should be addressed, including safety from further physical harm, hydration, food, sleep, hygiene, and education. Non-traumatic stressful

Box 14.1 Basic Objectives of Psychological First Aid (PFA)

- Establish a human connection in a non-intrusive, compassionate manner.
- Enhance immediate and ongoing safety, and provide physical and emotional comfort.
- Calm and orient emotionally overwhelmed or distraught survivors.
- Help survivors to articulate immediate needs and concerns, and gather additional information as appropriate.
- Offer practical assistance and information to help survivors address their immediate needs and concerns.
- Connect survivors as soon as possible to social support networks, including family members, friends, neighbors, and community helping resources.
- Support positive coping, acknowledge coping efforts and strengths, and empower survivors; encourage adults, children, and families to take an active role in their recovery.
- Provide information that may help survivors to cope effectively with the psychological impact of disasters.
- Facilitate continuity in disaster response efforts by clarifying how long the psychological first aid provider will be available. When appropriate, link the survivor to another member of a disaster response team or to indigenous recovery systems, mental health services, public-sector services, and organizations.

Sources: Fetter JC. Psychosocial response to mass casualty terrorism: guidelines for physicians. *Prim Care Companion to J Clin Psychiatry.* 2005;7(2):49–52; and Forbes D, Creamer MC, Phelps AJ, et al. Treating adults with acute stress disorder and post-traumatic stress disorder in general practice: a clinical update. *Med J Aust.* 2007;187:120–123.

---

stimuli should be minimized if possible. Excessive traumatic re-exposure especially through media coverage should be avoided. Social support will include facilitating the reconnection of survivors to natural communities such as schools, religious institutions, friends, and family. Parents and children in particular should be reunited as rapidly as possible if they had been separated. Psycho-education should be provided to survivors and their families to understand their emotions as normal reactions to extreme stress. Last, survivors and their families should be encouraged to find constructive activities, such as volunteering time,

Box 14.2 Overview of Psychological First Aid (PFA)

Preparing to Deliver Psychological First Aid

1. Entering the setting
2. Providing services
3. Maintaining a calm presence
4. Being sensitive to culture and diversity
5. Being aware of at-risk populations

Contact and Engagement

1. Introduce yourself
2. Ask about immediate needs

Safety and Comfort

1. Ensure immediate physical safety
2. Enhance sense of predictability, control, comfort, and safety
3. Provide simple information about disaster response activities and services
4. Attend to physical comfort
5. Promote social engagement
6. Attend to children who are separated from their parents
7. Protect from additional traumatic experiences and trauma reminders
8. Give special consideration for acutely bereaved individuals
9. Attend to the special needs of bereaved children and adolescents

Stabilization

1. Stabilization of emotionally overwhelmed survivors
2. Talking points for emotionally overwhelmed survivors
   Adults or caregivers
   Children and adolescents

Information Gathering:
Current Needs and Concerns

1. Nature and severity of experiences during the disaster
2. Death of a family member or close friend
3. Concerns about immediate post-disaster circumstances and ongoing threat
4. Separations from or concern about the safety of loved ones
5. Physical illness and need for medications

Continued on next page

Box 14.2 Continued

6. Losses incurred as a result of the disaster (home, school, neighborhood, business, personal property, or pets)
7. Extreme feelings of guilt or shame
8. Thoughts about causing harm to self or others
9. Lack of adequate supportive social network
10. Prior alcohol or drug use
11. Prior exposure to trauma and loss
12. Prior psychological problems
13. Specific youth, adult, and family concerns over developmental impact

Practical Assistance

1. Identify the most immediate need(s)
2. Clarify the need
3. Discuss an action plan
4. Act to address the need

Connection with Social Supports

1. Enhance access to primary support persons (family and significant others)
2. Encourage use of immediately available support persons
3. Discuss support seeking and giving
4. Help to identify external support, including professional help, when needed

Information on Coping

1. Provide basic information about stress reactions
2. Review common psychological reactions to traumatic experiences and losses
   Intrusive reactions
   Avoidance and withdrawal reactions
   Physical arousal reactions
   Trauma reminders
   Loss reminders
   Change reminders
   Hardships
   Grief reactions
   Traumatic grief
   Depression
   Physical reactions

---

3. Provide basic information on ways of coping
4. Demonstrate simple relaxation techniques
5. For parents or caregivers, review special considerations for children
   Assist with developmental issues
6. Assist with anger management
7. Address highly negative emotions
8. Help with sleep problems
9. Address substance abuse

Linkage with Collaborative Services

1. Provide direct link to additional needed services
2. Promote continuity in helping relationships

---

giving blood, take a cardiopulmonary resuscitation course class, and so forth. A return to routines should be promoted. Often in extreme stress, the ability to prioritize needs may be hampered. As such, disaster survivors should be supported in prioritizing problems, breaking them into reasonable and attainable tasks, and addressing them one at a time. Survivors should be educated about self-care strategies for stress such as relaxation techniques.

Conclusion

If you respond to disaster and mass casualty incidents, you will encounter a potentially large volume of patients with acute and diverse psychological reactions presenting for care. As such, all health providers should identify strategies to mitigate and minimize some of the adverse mental health consequences of such large-scale traumatic events. PFA has been identified as a paradigm for providing supportive early interventions including promoting a sense of safety and efficacy, education and normalization of reactions to acute stress, and connecting survivors with communities and services. While additional research is needed to continue to better understand the fluid and diverse nature of disasters and their impacts on communities, PFA will likely become the most evidence-based approach to promote both individual and community resiliency.

References

1. Watson PJ, Shalev AY. Assessment and treatment of adult acute responses to traumatic stress following mass traumatic events. *CNS Spectr.* 2005;10:123–131.

2. Hobfoll SE, Watson P, Bell CC, et al. Five essential elements of immediate and mid-term mass trauma intervention: empirical evidence. *Psychiatry.* 2007;70:283–315.

3. Everly GS Jr., Flynn BW. Principles and practical procedures for acute psychological first aid training for personnel without mental health experience. *Int J Emerg Ment Health.* 2006;8:93–100.

4. Watson P. Psychological first aid. In: Blumenfield M, Ursano RJ, Eds. *Interventions and Resilience After Mass Trauma.* Cambridge: Cambridge University Press; 2008.

5. Forbes D, Creamer MC, Phelps AJ, et al. Treating adults with acute stress disorder and post-traumatic stress disorder in general practice: a clinical update. *Med J Aust.* 2007;187:120–123.

6. NCTSN, NCPTSD, & MRC National Mental Health Work Group (2008). *Psychological First Aid for Medical Reserve Corps: Field Operations Guide.* Available at: **http://www.nctsn.org**, **www.ncptsd.org**, and **www.medical reservecorps.gov**. Accessed February 28, 2009.

7. Fetter JC. Psychosocial response to mass casualty terrorism: guidelines for physicians. *Prim Care Companion to J Clin Psychiatry.* 2005;7(2):49–52.

8. Hermann J, Cole V. *Psychological First Aid: Helping People Cope during Disasters and Public Health Emergencies. A Self-Study Program on Psychological First Aid and Workforce Resilience.* Rochester, NY: University of Rochester; 2006.

Understanding and Helping Responders

Craig L. Katz, MD

Mr. W is a 45-year-old married father of several young children and a member of the uniformed services who participated in the recovery of body parts at Ground Zero. He underwent a mental health evaluation in 2003 as part of a specialized program for World Trade Center responders and, although he appeared to be clinically depressed, denied having any problems and refused offers of treatment. Six months later, he called the evaluating social worker and agreed to enter treatment for a range of depressive and anxiety symptoms, even though he felt a deep sense of shame about the intensity of his emotions. Mr. W continues to receive combined medical treatment and psychotherapy in the program to address ongoing life stresses related to his work at Ground Zero as well as an unanticipated flood of memories related to childhood trauma.[1]

Responders' Place within the Disaster Community

Disaster responders like Mr. W are psychologically affected by a given event because of their membership in a "disaster community." The

- Responders occupy a vulnerable place near the center of the disaster community.

- External stresses of disaster work include pressurized expectations and witnessing death and destruction.

- Internal stresses of disaster work include grappling with role confusion, survivor guilt, and intense emotions.

- Engaging disaster workers around their psychological reactions to a disaster is crucial due to stigma surrounding mental health.

- A basic mental health screening should be incorporated into any physical health examination of responders.

disaster community consists of the people and organizations affected by disaster.[2] The original description of this concept derives from observations made following the 1985 crash of a chartered airline carrying elite United States Army members returning home to Fort Campbell, Kentucky, from an international peacekeeping mission (Figure 15.1).

Progressive circles of decreasing intensity of involvement emanate out from the central point of the direct victims, proceeding to the next of kin; to the service providers, including first responders; to support providers, including the local communities and others who support the

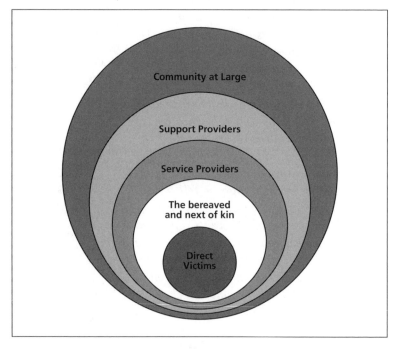

Figure 15.1 The disaster community based on an airplane that crashed en route to Fort Campbell, Kentucky, from Gander, Newfoundland, killing all 248 U.S. soldiers on board. Body identification occurred at Fort Campbell and Dover Air Force base.

Source: Wright KM, Ursano RJ, Bartone PT, Ingraham LH. The shared experience of catastrophe: an expanded classification of the disaster community. *Am J Orthopsychiatry.* 1990;60(1):35–42.

service providers like yourself; to the infrastructure within which the disaster response occurs. These circles of involvement may also span multiple communities, in this case the place of origin of the flight (Newfoundland), the destination of the flight (Fort Campbell), and the sites where body identification occurred (Fort Campbell and Dover Air Force Base).

The depiction of the disaster community graphically emphasizes how intensely exposed responders are by their position in the ring near the next of kin. Their psychological exposure to the disaster includes both physical and emotional factors. Unlike physical trauma with which you may be more acquainted from your health care practice, psychological trauma can be experienced even without physical proximity to a traumatic event. Emotional proximity may be just as important of a factor. For example, volunteer disaster workers working with the dead after an explosion on the *USS Iowa* were found to be more likely to have PTSD as well as other symptoms of distress if they identified with the deceased as a friend.[3] Responders are confronted with the double blow of physical and potential emotional exposure to a disaster.

The Stresses of Disaster Work

The physical and emotional proximity of responders to a disaster becomes reflected in the range of stressors they are exposed to.[4] External stressors include exposure to violent death and gruesome remains. Involvement in rescue and recovery efforts can be particularly stressful due to disturbing sensory experiences (e.g., sights and smells), the element of surprise involved in suddenly coming across a body, or exposure to the bodies of children. The mental health of morgue workers deserves special attention.[5] Other external sources of stress relate to having to deal with the anguish of next of kin and the pressurized work atmosphere characteristic of rescue and recovery efforts. Such pressure can lead responders to spend large amounts of time involved in rescue and recovery efforts, potentially exposing themselves to a longer duration of involvement than they can handle. In one study of over 28,000 rescue and recovery workers who like Mr. W participated in the response to the 9/11 attacks in New York City, duration of time spent at Ground Zero was a major predictor of who was likely to develop PTSD.[6] Some external stresses may even pre-date a disaster and relate to ongoing organizational stresses, such as labor relations issues.

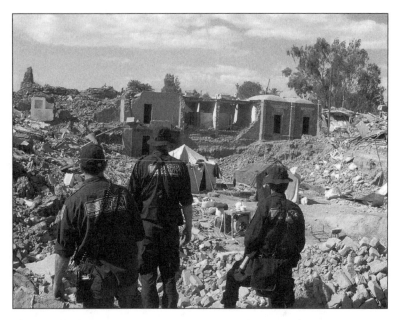

Figure 15.2 Rescue workers must each be confronted by a range of thoughts and feelings as they survey the aftermath of an earthquake in Bam, Iran.

Source: Courtesy of Jay Schnitzer, MD.

Internal experiences of a disaster can constitute other significant sources of stress for responders. In addition to the challenge of identifying with victims, responders may have to deal with a swirl of emotions surrounding unfamiliar experiences and of being confused about one's role or doubtful of one's ability to help or make a difference.[4] It can beget a lasting emotional pain to have felt lost or helpless while everyone else seemed to be running about purposefully and energetically at the scene of a disaster. And, like Mr. W, some responders may find that disaster work painfully and unexpectedly evokes memories of prior traumas, including childhood experiences or combat exposure. Survivor guilt can arise, especially if a responder has lost comrades or friends in the disaster. Identification, or overidentification, with victims may cause stress in responders. For instance, exposure to an injured child may lead a responder to identify that child with his own child and evoke guilt feelings should the child not survive.

Many people become involved in disaster response due to chance, such as hotel workers in the beachside resorts that suffered through the 2004 tsunami in Southeast Asia. The gulf that lies between coming to work prepared to work as a bartender and finding oneself rescuing drowning hotel guests poses an enormous stress on someone's ability to cope. Other responders are asked by their employers to perform disaster response work even though this lies outside of their usual job description. Following the 9/11 attacks in New York City, being asked to perform duties uncommon for one's job rendered responders more vulnerable to developing PTSD.[6] Crane operators know what it is like to work on a construction site but not what it is like to operate amid the death and destruction of Ground Zero.

Even being a hero can constitute a burden.[7] Disaster-stricken communities may need to believe in the heroism of someone in order to feel positive and secure as recovery proceeds, but few responders will be comfortable with the mantle of being a hero for long, if at all. This picture of themselves will all too often be at odds with their sense of not having saved enough people, of having just been doing their jobs, or of leading a personal life not at all as glorious or remarkable as their disaster work.

Being attuned to the range and types of responders and addressing their psychological needs, in collaboration with mental health personnel, is another task many primary care clinicians choose to do, or may be asked to do, on the disaster site. While not all clinicians may be comfortable with this task and may have limited training, there is special meaning and support when a respected clinician empathizes with the psychological needs of responders while providing medical services.

Addressing the Psychological Needs of Responders

Helping disaster responders cope with the emotions of their experience starts with helping them to become aware of the psychological challenges they face. They may need your assistance with recognizing, accepting, and seeking help for their emotions. The disaster response community is largely male, and, for this reason, not often pre-disposed to seek out mental health care. The first responder community in particular is often steeped in a nearly religious faith; the community believes that participation in a psychological debriefing session is all it needs. It is not typical for patients like Mr. W, who are ashamed of how they are feeling, to take time to come for treatment. One sam-ple of 9/11 responders found that only 3% had seen a mental health professional prior to participating in a 9/11 mental health screening.[8] Yet, the intensity and discomfort of emotions unleashed by exposure to a disaster make it all the more troubling when responders minimize their emotional lives in the ways they did before the event.

Having access to mental health care is therefore crucial for disaster responders, potentially helping them deal with the residual effects of their disaster work and possibly even with unmet pre-disaster mental health needs underscored by the event. Health care professionals not identified with the mental health field are in a unique position to improve this access. Perhaps even more so than with people in general, disaster responders are far more likely to complain of aches and pains to you as an internist or family physician than to complain to a psychiatrist or other mental health professional of psychic pain.

You should conduct at least a rudimentary mental health screening of every responder with whom you have a clinical contact after a recent disaster exposure. Methods for screening for common disaster-related problems such as PTSD, major depression, and alcohol problems are described elsewhere in this book (see Chapter 8). You may even find that discussing smoking cessation with these patients paves the way for a discussion of their mental well-being. Identifying a reason for concern for a responder's mental health then leads to the crucial step of engaging them in care, whether with you or with a mental health colleague. Co-locating your medical practice with mental health professionals in the post-disaster setting (and even under normal circumstances) can help to reduce obstacles to pursuing a mental health referral.[1]

Your success in convincing responders that they can and should address their mental health can be aided by a number of clinical approaches. (See Box 15.1.) First, it may be necessary to "de-psychologize," "medicalize," or normalize their symptoms as much as is possible. This can be accomplished by emphasizing the underlying biology of disorders like PTSD (e.g., too much stress hormone or adrenalin) or

Box 15.1   Understanding and Helping Responders: Clinical Approaches

---

- Normalize symptoms if possible.
- Focus on function, not feelings.
- Consider medications or psychotherapy.

---

emphasizing problems most people can acknowledge needing help with (e.g., insomnia or poor concentration). Second, feelings or emotions need not be the focus of a discussion about mental health. Instead, consider focusing on how the worker appears to be functioning at a lower than usual level in his work or family life since the event. Third, most disaster-related conditions can be treated with medications or psychotherapy. Gauging your patient's relative comfort, or aversion, for one or the other modality can help identify a comfortable starting place for treatment (e.g., "I understand you are against medications, but how about then just going for some talking therapy?"). Fourth, asking patients to at least go for an evaluation or consultation with a mental health professional rather than treatment can help to initiate a step-wise approach to getting help. Finally, many workers prefer to get help from mental health resources that are not associated with their employer, especially when issues of "fitness for duty" may arise.

Your goal in taking these approaches with disaster responders is not necessarily for them to see a mental health professional or to accept a psychotropic prescription but rather to address their mental health for their own good and that of their family through any healthy means. Many people, and especially responders, can rely on a range of all-important sources of social support in dealing with the burden of disaster work. These include informal exchanges with family, friends, co-workers, and the clergy. Formalized peer assistance programs such as those that exist for New York City police officers also have a role.[9] The key is for responders, such as Mr. W, to possess or develop facility with acknowledging and sharing how they are feeling, possibly with you as their primary care provider, often with a mental health professional, but always with someone. Sometimes getting to this point may even constitute the goal of your clinical intervention.

References

1. Katz CL, Smith RP, Silverton M, Holmes A, Bravo C, Jones K, et al. A mental health program for Ground Zero rescue and recovery workers: cases and observations. *Psychiatric Services.* 2006;57(9):1335–1338.

2. Wright KM, Ursano RJ, Bartone PT, Ingraham LH. The shared experience of catastrophe: an expanded classification of the disaster community. *Am J Orthopsychiatry.* 1990;60(1):35–42.

3. Ursano RJ, Fullerton CS, Vance K, Kao TC. Post-traumatic stress disorder and identification in disaster workers. *Am J Psychiatry.* 1999;156:353–359.

4. Disaster Psychiatry Outreach. *The Essentials of Disaster Psychiatry: A Training Course for Mental Health Professionals.* New York, NY: Disaster Psychiatry Outreach; 2008.

5. Merlino JP. The Other Ground Zero. In: Pandya A, Katz C, Eds. *Disaster Psychiatry: Intervening When Nightmares Come True.* Hillsdale, NJ: Analytic Press; 2004:31–36.

6. Perrin MA, DiGrande L, Wheeler K, Thorpe L, Farfel M, Brackbill R. Differences in PTSD prevalence and associated risk factors among World Trade Center rescue and recovery workers. *Am J Psychiatry.* 2007;9:1385–1394.

7. Goren E. Society's use of the hero following a national trauma. *Am J Psychoanalysis.* 2007;67:7–52.

8. Smith RP, Katz CL, Holmes A, Herbert R, Levin S, Moline J, et al. Mental health status of World Trade Center rescue and recovery workers and volunteers: New York City, July 2002. *Morbidity and Mortality Weekly Report.* 2004;53(35):812–815.

9. Dowling FG, Moynihan G, Genet B, Lewis J. A peer-based assistance program for officers with the New York City Police Department: report of the effects of Sept. 11, 2001. *Am J Psychiatry.* 2006;163(1):151–153.

Social Interventions in Disaster

Todd F. Holzman, MD

Peter, greeting an arriving cross-country evacuation flight of Katrina hurricane survivors, observes Asian family members holding each other, appearing quite distressed. They had no idea where they had landed. Their 8-year-old daughter was anxiously holding onto her mother who was herself distraught, frightened, and near tears. Her father appeared sad, downcast, and passive. With daughter translating, parents vividly recalled their horrors and terror as well as the graft and corruption they experienced before immigrating from Southeast Asia. Hearing their stories allowed Peter to realistically discuss their situation, soothe their anxieties, and enabled them to shape more realistic expectations. The support of eight state and non-governmental organizations provided tangible, emotional, and community support, including health, housing, school, employment, community, and religious connections. Five days later, he saw the mother's eyes well up with joy, watching her daughter board a small yellow school bus, beaming in her new clothes and book bag.

- Disasters disrupt interpersonal and societal connections, leaving survivors feeling helpless and forgotten.
- Social influences contributing to disasters shape survivors' responses.
- Preparations to provide social interventions are essential.
- Within social groups reassurance and managing expectations are essential.
- It is important to reduce the social stigma of mental health services and try to make them more acceptable.
- Quarantines and isolation present special social problems.
- It is helpful to anticipate a lingering post-disaster period of disillusionment and discouragement.
- As time passes, isolation subsides, social networks regroup, stories are shared, connections strengthen, and healing may occur.

131

Disasters Disrupt Interpersonal and Societal Connections

Disasters are social occurrences that terrifyingly disrupt and rupture interpersonal and societal connections. Survivors feel helpless, isolated, alone, and forgotten. Whether fearing or sustaining injury, abandonment, mutilation, or death, each feels at the mercy of a person, group, or situation that has no mercy. The individual is overwhelmed and at risk of losing her normal coping skills. The compassionate presence of another person who is there to help can be an antidote. This chapter will look at post-disaster vulnerability and areas where health professionals can promote individual and community resilience and recovery through social interventions.[1] When the clinician is not providing the intervention himself, he can still provide direction or support to promote social interventions facilitating recovery.

Causes of Disasters Influence Survivors' Responses

Disasters may be caused by natural calamities, epidemics, and by accidents, such as an industrial release of toxin, or an air, sea, or land transportation vehicle crash. They also may be purposefully malicious, such as an act of war, terrorism, a school shooting, personal torture, or genocide. A survivor's response is influenced by the social factors involved. Evil intention exacerbates the situation because victims and survivors have been targeted by the perpetrators. In seeking to respond to survivors' needs, interventions need to address these social factors.

Social Planning and Practiced Preparations Enhance Disaster Response

Social and public health disaster preparations range from safe building codes to stockpiled medications and vaccines, to plans for operational continuity for airport security, correctional facilities, and business and financial institutions. It is crucial for schools to have disaster plans, including training for teachers and counselors. Other essential social preparations include training emergency responders and health care personnel, development of hospital surge capacity, and planning and updating action plans for facilities and public agencies, especially inter-agency command, control, communications, and structures (see Chapters 2 and 12).

First Responders Assume Important Conflicting Roles

Initial responders strive to bring social order to the disaster scene. Their goal is to establish safety, organize initial triage, care for the injured, and provide for survivors' basic needs. Health workers consistently volunteer in disaster situations.

Large numbers of people are required to help in disasters. Airport simulated crash drills at Boston's Logan Airport involve more than 100 distinct agencies and groups.[2] Social preparation in such drills involves identifying those essential functions each agency or business is responsible for, then having instruction, information, and cross-training for those functions that must carry on over the time of the disaster in a chain of command succession. Advance training allows responders to establish social relationships, making their future work together more effective under the stress of a disaster.

Community response to a disaster is often effective and may be strikingly heroic. Communities tend to initially pull together—with individuals and groups helping each other with selfless bravery, mutual care, respect, and concern. Later, this behavior may return to "usual" social discriminations, sometimes with a venting of frustration and animosity for any perceived unfairness and disappointment in the disaster response.

Essential responders, themselves disaster survivors, experience conflicting personal and professional demands, which may set up impossible choices. While facing community expectations to respond professionally, responders simultaneously desire to seek safety and care for their own families. Communication and infrastructure disruptions and contagion risks may isolate responders from their work or from their families. Your traditional social role as a health care professional is to continue your professional work during disasters (see Chapter 3).

Communication and Reassurance: Managing Expectations

The social organization and coordination of disaster response are enhanced by drills, which rehearse the operations of the command structure. Drills and practice teach and reinforce the use of protocols for mobilization of rapid social interventions to provide safety and security; medical and psychological services, basic food, shelter, and clothing; identification, tracking, and communication among survivors; and news and informational briefings.[3]

At the scene, social and individual shock and the impact of the situation are mitigated by orientation and information, reassurance and safety, identification, expectations for care, and especially the continuing, compassionate presence of helpers. The established command structure and organization should enable identification, registration, and tracking of survivors and ways to communicate with their families and friends, including private places that do not interfere with other emergency activities. These places must be large enough to accommodate all those present at the scene. Since there is enough chaos on disaster scenes, it is optimal not to increase it by crowding anxious and upset people into small spaces. Therefore, in order to facilitate social cohesion, designated areas for patients and family communication outside the emergency treatment area need to be made available.

Care of Families of Those Who Have Died

Since death is often a consequence of disasters and may affect large numbers of people, it is important to anticipate the need for bereavement care and information for the relatives and friends of those who are either terminal casualties of the disaster or of those who did not survive (see Chapter 13). Friends and relatives need clear information about the nature of the patient's problems and treatments, to be allowed to see the survivor or the victim's body, and to receive responses to their questions. Their needs and reactions should be respected, as should sensitivities to their cultural and religious traditions, which can seem strange to a visiting disaster volunteer. Sensitive responses from clinicians are often recalled with gratitude. Survivors often turn to religion, faithfully seeking their God. As the old soldier observed, "There are no atheists in a foxhole."

Quarantine and Isolation Present Special Problems

It was estimated about half the target population in Singapore fled from SARS before quarantine could be established.[4] In Canada during the SARS scare, remaining at home with family allowed for more mutual support and timely requests for medical attention.[4] Family reluctance to separate from each other, as well as other people's fear and the social stigma of contamination by the victim, creates serious social conflict for clinicians. Social pressures to attend patriotic assemblies and parades during WWI were associated with high contagion of influenza pandemic. Clinicians must convey clear, factual information about the risks of such large assemblies, and benefits of required isolation and quarantine. They should present, in collaboration with public safety officers, the real risks to health and security.

Post-Disaster Disillusionment and Discouragement

As the acute crisis ameliorates, the novelty wears off, the initial hopes for a rapid return to normal fade, the losses remain, and the shock becomes an undeniable reality. In addition, the media attention fades and volunteers go home. It is helpful to anticipate a period of lingering disillusionment and discouragement that often follows.

As seen following recent disasters in New Orleans, Burma, China, Thailand, and elsewhere, the destruction of villages and communities, the relocation and homelessness, and the sudden inability to work and provide sustenance and safety for their families comprise a new reality for survivors. Ruins, blighted landscapes, and flooded former residences are constant reminders. Mutual irritability between survivors and helpers, anger and disappointment, a sense of ineffectiveness, and frustration and exhaustion may soon dominate social interactions. You should anticipate these reactions. Allot time for interventions that allow for the expression of these emotions, with calm recognition of the necessary rebuilding of relationships and social structures that provide renewed connections and strength.

Social networks, lifelong relationships, religious institutions, work, health care, and community and government organizations are part of the fabric of life disrupted by a disaster. The individuals' responses are primarily supported by this social network. In poor inner-city or isolated rural settings, the efforts of disaster responders may not be sought out because these "helpers" have long been viewed with suspicion or distrust as outsiders or government officials or there may be some unique cultural or personal stigma. Responders' assumptions about such specific issues are often misinformed. Collaboration with both official and local community leaders can build trust and help focus energy on problems they care about and on effective solutions.

Healing Occurs as Time Passes and Connections Strengthen

A disaster, now part of communal history, is never forgotten, but basic resilience and social reorientation provide avenues for post-disaster recovery. Time and gradual healing may allow for more realistic and effective reconstruction, relocation, and social reorientation to life's new realities. Isolation subsides, social networks regroup, and stories are shared repeatedly. Anniversaries, memorials, and the retelling of personal experiences continue. For some, symptoms of post-traumatic stress disorder interfere, though in most cases these resolve with time and treatment. Survivors helping others, or volunteering in altruistic efforts, may increase their personal sense of self-esteem and effectiveness. Healing is further enhanced by social interventions such as reestablishing traditional family, cultural, and religious practices.

Community meetings, advocacy groups, and grassroots organizations may be encouraged and created by survivors to focus on the issues they share, obstacles they face, and challenges they feel. These groups and meetings have proven effective in directing reconstruction efforts. Survivors working at the grassroots level with both officials and the media, mutually seeking resolution of communal problems, promote a healthy sense of well-being and efficacy for all involved. As basic resilience takes over, isolation subsides, and personal and social connections are eventually re-established, most survivors will be able to integrate their new reality. Social interventions described in this chapter are designed to ameliorate the most horrific aspects of the disaster and its aftermath.

References

1. Kaniasty K, Norris FH. Social support in the aftermath of disasters, catastrophes, and acts of terrorism: altruistic, overwhelmed, uncertain, antagonistic, and patriotic communities. In: Ursano RJ, Norwood AE, Fullerton CS, Eds. *Bioterrorism: Psychological and Public Health Interventions.* Cambridge: Cambridge University Press; 2004:200–231.

2. Holzman TF, Stoddard FJ. Since 1998, Drs. Holzman and Stoddard have participated, together with over 100 agencies, in disaster drills at Logan International Airport, Boston.

3. Hobfoll SE. Guiding community intervention following terrorist attack. In: Neria Y, Gross R, Marshall R, Susser E, Eds. *9/11: Mental Health in the Wake of Terrorist Attacks.* Cambridge: Cambridge University Press; 2006:215–230.

4. Pitch RF. Hospital as a Patient Care Provider: Patient Care Strategies II. In: Shultz JM, Espinel Z, Cohen RE, Insignares JR, Rosenfeld L, Flynn BW, et al., Eds. Disaster Behavioral Health Awareness Training for Health Care Professionals, 2004. Syllabus. University of Miami School of Medicine, Miami, Florida, 2004

Psychological Interventions

Frederick J. Stoddard, Jr., MD

Peter worked with Mary, a nurse practitioner, in a clinic that responded to a terrible explosion in an iron foundry. The clinic provided care to several survivors, although many died in the blast. Peter referred Arthur, a 36-year-old survivor, to Mary for counseling. Mary had some training in cognitive therapy. The survivor was seen due to his wife's concern about his withdrawal at home for over 3 months after recovery from minor burns to his arms and cheek. He lost one friend in the explosion, and another was injured. Clinical evaluation indicated grief over the loss of his friend, insomnia, re-experiencing of the blast, and fear for his life. He was thinking of not returning to work. He was eager to recover his good health. Mary explained the course of normal grieving and that he had post-traumatic stress disorder, which was helpful to know for him and his wife. He was glad to learn that these symptoms usually taper over time and that people who return to work often cope better than those who don't. He agreed to see Mary in follow-up sessions with the supportive involvement of his wife. Over 3 months he came back for five

- The scope of psychological interventions is broad and includes all steps that promote psychological well-being.

- Principles of psychological interventions include promoting a sense of safety, calming, a sense of self and community efficacy, connectedness, and hope.

- Psychological interventions should begin before a disaster and continue for years after.

- These interventions are usually more effective than medications.

- Interventions include preventive triage, individual, family, and group therapies for distress, PTSD, phobias, depression, and substance abuse.

- Follow-up and referral for long-term interventions identify and may help those whose symptoms persist or worsen.

sessions that seemed to relieve his grieving and to reinforce his positive attitude about return to work and reconnecting with friends. He was able to talk about his sadness, to recognize irrational fears about work, and to venture out from home. With Mary's empathic encouragement, he returned to visit the foundry, recognized that new safety measures had reduced the dangers, and was reassured to see that others were now back at work. With gradual lessening of his feelings of grief and anxiety, he successfully returned to work. From this, Peter realized that incorporating aspects of Mary's psychological intervention into his care of disaster victims would not be too hard.

Overview

Like Mary, many clinicians are intuitively empathic and interpersonally responsive, and may find what follows to be like the character who discovered he was speaking prose without knowing it![1] If you are already using techniques described here, this chapter may help strengthen the basis for your psychologically informed practice. Primary care clinicians are often the first to intervene psychologically after disasters. This chapter provides an overview of these interventions and ways to use them. Early triage and assessment identify strengths, vulnerabilities, and social supports. Since most affected people are resilient and cope well, psychological reinforcement of strengths such as practical coping skills, bravery, altruism, and compassion is helpful. Interventions also should identify needed social supports and seek to remedy them.

Why Psychological Interventions?

While medications tend to be easier and quicker interventions to prescribe, psychological interventions are often more effective than medications in intervening for distress related to disasters and in treating psychological disorders due to post-traumatic stress.

Types of Psychological Interventions

Psychological interventions refer here to the elements of the principal clinical interventions to lessen distress, which can be used or adapted by primary care clinicians after disasters. The primary objectives are to benefit patients, but some of them may also help families, groups, communities, and organizations. While nearly all interventions are outpatient, some patients require hospitalization for psychiatric or substance abuse treatment. While psychological interventions are the major intervention for nearly all patients, they overlap with *psychopharmacological interventions* where the target symptoms are mainly psychological. Many patients who will receive medications will also receive psychological interventions. They overlap also with *social interventions* whose main objectives are for populations. Psychological interventions may occur before disasters and may present acutely or in the long-term post-acute phase of disasters.

Goals

Psychological interventions are all those steps with the goal of benefiting the psychological well-being of those impacted by disasters. While they are an important part of clinical treatments in primary care, they aren't limited to this. Most preventive and early interventions are public health interventions. They are not treatments but rather steps for everyone whose goal is to enhance coping, foster resilience, and assist the most impacted individuals in receiving screening, medical evaluation, or treatment.[2] Within this broad definition, *psychological first aid* (PFA) and *social interventions* are two kinds of mostly non-clinical psychological intervention and are discussed earlier in this section of the book. The goal of this chapter is to present *clinical* psychological interventions useful for primary care clinicians to know about, and hopefully use, in the context of disasters.

Earlier chapters address assessment, ways to triage patients, to screen them, to identify which people, and what problems require clinical evaluation to be sure they are safe and not a danger to self or others, and to recognize bereavement. Once you have identified patients needing psychological help, what can you do? What if you "don't feel good" about someone you see who is impacted by a disaster? How do you manage a patient you identify as threatening, dangerous, or intoxicated? What clinical psychological interventions can work in the disaster setting? This chapter begins to address these questions.

Standard clinical psychological interventions to reduce distress and calm the patient include understanding how the disaster has affected her, assessing specific areas of concern, and responding to these concerns *over time*. Stepped intervention programs, such as will be described later, provide psychologically informed interventions appropriate to the stage of care that the patient is in, something like physical therapy interventions modified gradually from when a patient is bedridden, to beginning to ambulate, to when she can participate in more strenuous stretching, strengthening, and conditioning.[3] All medical interventions should be psychologically informed from preparatory trainings, to early phase, acute phase, and long-term interventions seeking to relieve bereavement and to support recovery.[4]

Clinical psychological interventions should be geared to identified concerns and needs of the population. For instance, for those with injuries, the interventions that are most helpful are beginning to be understood. In one study, most concerns of injured patients were with aspects of physical health (68%), work, and finances (59%), while only about 25% of concerns were psychological.[5] This suggests that early psychological interventions for injured adults should usually focus on supporting physical recovery, work, and finances, as Mary's interventions did, whereas for children and adolescents the focus is more on pain and stress, physical recovery, family support, and school.[6]

Early Interventions

Historically, from World War II, it was thought that group debriefing following battle stress was an optimal psychological intervention to reduce psychological stress and return soldiers to action. While it has many forms, psychological debriefing soon after a major stressful experience refers to a single or a few sessions with a group or individual, carried out usually but not necessarily by a mental health professional. It usually includes encouraging people to tell their story of what happened, asking how they felt, teaching about future reactions, and suggesting ways of coping. This practice has been found in multiple randomized controlled studies to cause more harm than good with long-term findings that some people react to this with increased stress.[7] Although still advocated by some, psychological debriefing is not recommended. However, operational debriefing remains of value. It is used when first responders such as fire fighters, or others with well-defined roles in assigned operations, report on progress in achieving tasks assigned to them. Evidence-informed early interventions are described in Tables 17.1 and 17.2.[7]

Although all approaches to early intervention utilize brief education and advice, the most stressed individuals may be so anxious and confused as to not be able to make sense of this form of help, and clinical psychological interventions based on the preceding psychological assumptions and targets may be needed.

How can the seven targets in Table 17.2 be useful in care provided by you as a primary care clinician? First, to increase therapeutic exposure to the stimuli associated with the trauma seems illogical and is what the patient fears most. However, Mary's empathically helping her patient revisit the foundry, for example—controlled re-experiencing and re-exposure, lessened his fears and was a key step in his return to work.

Psychological Interventions

 Table 17.1 Assumptions about Early Interventions

1. Most people will recover.
2. It is important to intervene soon after the trauma.
3. It is important to normalize acute stress reactions.
4. Brief interventions will be adequate for most survivors.
5. It is important to focus on the survivor's ongoing adaptive coping.
6. It is important to offer social support.
7. It is important to provide active outreach to survivors.
8. It is vital to identify high-risk survivors.

 Table 17.2 Targets for Early Interventions

1. Increase therapeutic exposure to the stimuli associated with the trauma (exposure therapy).
2. Modify negative trauma-related beliefs.
3. Improve coping efforts possibly by reducing high arousal or by reducing fear of acute stress reactions.
4. Prevent maladaptive coping (e.g., extreme avoidance or social isolation/alcohol/drugs).
5. Increase social support.
6. Prevent loss of resources and reduce continuing negative consequences.
7. Maintain functioning soon after the trauma.

Modifying trauma-related negative beliefs is part of the stepwise therapeutic process. The clinician improves the patient's coping by encouraging mastery of specific PTSD symptoms, such as by reinforcing positive thoughts that the patient can succeed in reducing hyper-arousal symptoms, and in turn, reduce their fear of an acute stress response. Positive recovery is further reinforced by actively discouraging maladaptive behaviors, such as social isolation or substance abuse, and encouraging increased friendships and social support. The clinician's interest and actions to prevent loss of resources (food, shelter, etc.) further prevent negative emotional consequences of disaster. And, last, maintaining functioning whether as a contributing family member, student, or worker is a goal of all the prior steps and can lead to sustained recovery from PTSD.

In considering early or acute interventions, some psychodynamic perspectives were provided by psychiatrists in training in New York, who founded Disaster Psychiatry Outreach (DPO). DPO responded to the crash of SwissAir Flight 111 in 1998, EgyptAir 990, 9/11, and other disasters. The DPO reflected on psychodynamic meanings of psychiatric work in the context of disasters.[8] Among its observations was the concept of a "trauma tent"—how its presence was experienced among survivors and workers after disasters. This represented an "invisible" collaboration, and likely idealization, which "seemed to put others at ease" indicated by the many emergency and relief workers who knew the members by name and pager number. The trauma tent bears a resemblance to one of the seminal contributions by the British pediatrician and psychoanalyst D.W. Winnicott's, the "holding environment," which permits the healing work of psychotherapy. He derived this concept from his idea of how the mother's nurturance enabled the development of the infant's separate self, analogous to how the caring clinician in a disaster creates an empathic interpersonal environment within which a patient may become aware of healing psychologically after emotional and physical trauma. In another reflection, the New York group commented helpfully on countertransference reactions in mental health professionals working in disasters. They stated, "Not everybody is suited to disaster response, and this is especially the case when the responder is acting more out of their needs than those of the survivors." Such reflections may be of interest to primary care clinicians as well, as they strive to provide compassionate psychological care in disasters.

Recommendations for Planning Psychological Interventions After Disasters

A consensus conference of experts in the field of psychological responses to disasters identified five essential elements for early and mid-term mass trauma interventions based on empirical evidence.[9] The elements orient the clinician to psychologically informed interventions for all ages and point to skills for which further education is available. The five elements are promoting

1. A sense of safety
2. Calming, including interventions such as those by Mary
3. A sense of self and community efficacy like Mary's patient's return to work
4. A connectedness such as resuming socializing with friends
5. Hope

Long-Term Clinical Psychological Interventions

It is useful to be aware that a range of psychiatric and psychological therapies is available in most Western countries for longer term disaster-related mental health problems. As the acute phase gives way to the longer term, psychological first aid, group support, and brief counseling are done by all health service providers. Clinical counseling and psychotherapy may be provided by all mental health professionals. In Western countries, you may choose to refer some patients for common available psychological treatments. Among these are short-term therapy, psychodynamic therapy, family therapy, developmentally targeted play therapy for children, parent counseling, group therapy, geriatric therapy, long-term psychodynamic psychotherapy, medication groups for the seriously and persistently mentally ill, and substance abuse programs.[10]

The evidence base for treatments after early interventions is strongest for cognitive behavior therapy or CBT, including for children, and consists of varying types of short-term interventions.[11,12] Cognitive therapy was developed to treat depression and anxiety and has been adapted for PTSD.[13,14] Its goal is to teach the patient to identify and to logically challenge irrational beliefs that may influence his response to a situation and lead to negative emotion and to decide whether the belief is helpful and whether to change it. Exposure therapy for PTSD entails imaginal exposure or verbal recounting of the traumatic memory, followed by *in vivo* exposure to the feared object, situation, or memory, such as Arthur's return to his workplace or a soldier being sent back onto the battlefield, with the goal of evoking memory and excessive anxiety associated with the traumatic experience, and promoting eventual habituation and processing of the traumatic memory. It may include relaxation training.[15] Prolonged exposure includes psycho-education, discussion, and processing following the imaginal exposure to the traumatic memory.[16] Stress inoculation training for PTSD is education about trauma-related symptoms together with methods of managing anxiety such as relaxation training, cognitive restructuring, thought-stopping, role-playing, and assertiveness training.

The Threatening, Dangerous, or Intoxicated Patient

While such patients were discussed earlier, this is the first discussion of treatment for threatening, dangerous, or intoxicated patients. Identification of such patients is the first step. Ongoing consultation with mental health personnel is helpful in anticipating these issues and developing optimal options for intervention over time. If the patient is threatening or dangerous, before proceeding with medical care, security personnel or other helpers may need to be called upon to ensure one's own and others' safety. Once that is ensured, further history may be obtained to learn what has triggered the patient's upset. Even for those with clear disaster-related emotional trauma, concurrent physical causes should be considered such as substance abuse, medications, brain injury, infection, and so forth. While this is being clarified, psychological interventions can help calm the patient over time. In some cases, and when possible, psychopharmacological intervention with an anxiolytic or antipsychotic may aid management of disturbed patients. When someone worsens rather than calms, it may be best to move her, if possible, to an acute care, substance abuse, or inpatient psychiatric setting for further evaluation and treatment.

Conclusion

Psychological interventions include a range of interventions spanning the early and long-term periods after a disaster. Among the principles informing the primary care clinician's psychological approaches in the context of disaster is promoting a sense of safety, calming, a sense of self, and community efficacy, connectedness, and hope. The psychological intervention by Peter's associate, Mary, a nurse practitioner, introduces the broader range of interventions for treating or empathically alleviating the suffering of your patients due to post-traumatic stress disorder. It may be useful to integrate some elements of her interventions into your practices. Ongoing consultation with mental health personnel is helpful in triage, choice of treatments, and identification of complicated cases. Psychological interventions after trauma are often the most effective of all interventions.

References

1. Moliere. *Le Bourgeois Gentilhomme.* Act II, Scene IV; 1670.

2. Charney DS. Psychobiological mechanisms of resilience and vulnerability: implications for successful adaptation to extreme stress. *Am J Psychiatry.* 2004;161:195–216.

3. Zatzick D. Collaborative care for injured victims of individual and mass trauma: a health services research approach to developing early interventions. In: Ursano RJ, Fullerton CS, Norwood AE, Eds. *Terrorism and Disaster: Individual and Community Mental Health Interventions.* Cambridge: Cambridge University Press; 2003:189–205.

4. Zatzick DF, Russo J, Rajotte E, Uehara E, Roy-Byrne P, Ghesquiere A, et al. Strengthening the patient-provider relationship in the aftermath of physical trauma through an understanding of the nature and severity of post-traumatic concerns. *Psychiatry.* 2007;70(3):260–273.

5. Stoddard FJ. Care of infants, children and adolescents with burn injuries. In: Lewis M, Ed. *Child and Adolescent Psychiatry.* 3rd ed. Philadelphia: Lippincott Williams & Wilkins; 2002:1188–1208.

6. Stoddard FJ, Saxe G. Ten-year research review of physical injuries. *J Am Acad Child Adolesc Psychiatry.* 2001;40(10):1128–1145.

7. Rose S, Bisson J, Churchill R, Wessely S. Psychological debriefing for post-traumatic stress disorder (PTSD). The Cochrane Library 2002; Issue 2, Art No: CD 000560. DOI:10.10023/14651858.

8. Katz CL, Nathaniel R. Disasters, psychiatry, and psychodynamics. *J Am Acad Psychoanalysis.* 2002;30(4):519–529.

9. Hobfoll SE, Watson P, Bell CC, Bryant RA, Brymer MJ, Friedman MJ, et al. Five essential elements in immediate and mid-term mass trauma intervention: empirical evidence. *Psychiatry.* 2007;70(4):283–315.

10. Schechter D, Coates SW. Relationally and developmentally focused interventions with young children and their caregivers in the wake of terrorism and other violent experiences. In: Neria Y, Gross R, Marshall R, Eds. *9/11: Mental Health in the Wake of Terrorist Attacks.* Cambridge: Cambridge University Press; 2006:402–423.

11. March JS, Amaya-Jackson L, Murray MC, Schulte A. Cognitive-behavioral psychotherapy for children and adolescents with post-traumatic stress disorder after a single incident stressor. *J Am Acad Child Adolesc Psychiatry.* 1998;37:586–593.

12. Cohen JA, Mannarino AP, Perel JM, Staron V. A pilot randomized controlled trial of combined trauma-focused CBT and sertraline for childhood PTSD symptoms. *J Am Acad Child Adolesc Psychiatry.* 2007;46(7):811–819.

13. Beck AT, Emery G, Greenberg RL. *Anxiety Disorders and Phobias: A Cognitive Perspective.* New York, NY: Basic Books; 1985.

14. Marks I, Lovell K, Noshirvani IH, Livanou M, Thrasher S. Treatment of post-traumatic stress disorder by exposure and/or cognitive restructuring. *Arch General Psychiatry.* 1998;55:317–325.

15. Keane TM, Zimmering RT, Caddell JM. A behavioral formulation of PTSD in Vietnam veterans. *Behav Ther.* 1985;8:9–12.

16. Foa EB, Dancu CV, Hembree EA, Jaycox LH, Meadows EA, Street G. The efficacy of exposure therapy, stress inoculation training, and their combination in ameliorating PTSD for female victims of assault. *J Consult & Clin Psychol.* 1999;67:194–200.

Psychopharmacology

Kristina Jones, MD

Susan, a nurse who is a friend of yours, approaches you on the third day after a disaster and says that she is "losing it." She has not slept in 3 days, is irritable, forgetful, and cannot concentrate. She says that she had taken sertraline in the past for anxiety, and she is afraid that if she leaves the hospital she will relapse on alcohol, from which she has been sober for 3 years. She is about to go home because the relief nurses are coming to replace her. She asks you for a sleep medication. What interventions

- The evidence base for acute psychopharmacological interventions in disasters is weak.
- A medical history, including psychiatric history, should be taken and a physical examination done.
- Biological factors affecting the absorption, metabolism, distribution, and excretion of medication should be considered. The history of medication allergy, adverse reactions, potential drug interactions, and substance abuse should be evaluated.
- Physical injury is a risk factor for later anxiety and posttraumatic stress.
- The goals of psychopharmacological treatment are to reduce symptoms, typically

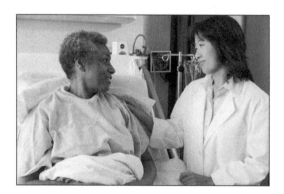

Figure 18.1 Anxiety and insomnia are the most common emergency room presentations in the acute post-disaster stage.

Source: ©Monkey Business Images/Dreamstime.com

(Continued next page.)

Continued from previous page.

anxiety, shock, insomnia, depression, or agitation that may interfere with coping after the disaster, and to minimize risk of adverse effects.

- Common diagnoses are acute and post-traumatic stress disorder, major depression, alcohol withdrawal, and, less commonly, mania and drug-induced psychoses.

- While for children and adolescents the principles of pediatric psychopharmacology after a disaster are similar to those for adults, developmental factors are central in assessment and diagnosis, in considerations about metabolism and growth, in dosing based on body weight, and in identifying target symptoms and adverse drug effects.

are useful? You might give a prescription for sertraline 50 mg for 14 days until she can follow-up with a psychiatrist. Or you might prescribe lorazepam 0.5 mg po qhs, dispensing five (5) tablets. Suggest that she also drop by her local Alcoholics Anonymous meeting.

Psychopharmacology in the acute phase of disasters focuses on addressing symptoms that may impair a patient's ability to cope with each stage of disaster. This may include anxiety or shock in the immediate aftermath, insomnia in the days and weeks that follow, or clinical depression in the months afterward. There are few well-designed placebo-controlled trials for acute intervention. Instead, you must intervene for specific target symptoms following common principles from primary care, emergency, and consultation psychiatry medicine. In the United States, while primary care clinicians prescribe the majority of psychopharmacological drugs for children and adults, you are unlikely to have experience with prescribing in disaster settings.

In the first week after a disaster, primary care clinicians are often called upon to address anxiety and insomnia, and, in treating the physically injured, may be the first to examine patients with the uncommon presentations of acute psychiatric disorders, such as panic, dissociation, or psychosis.

In the post-acute phase, after 4 to 8 weeks, patients present with more apparent groups of symptoms that are recognizable as psychiatric syndromes such as panic disorder, major depression, and post-traumatic stress disorder.

Medical Evaluation

History

Relevant issues for psychotropic prescribing from your patient's history include any history of toxic, infectious, or radioactive exposure, head injury, seizure, cardiac, or respiratory problems, as well as specific injuries arising from the disaster such as lacerations or burns. Also assess psychiatric history for prior diagnoses and treatment. Evaluate medications current and past, and possible alcohol and substance use/abuse. If time allows, ask about legal issues, school or work, family, developmental risk due to age, and with women, possible pregnancy. Particular attention should be paid to systemic illness, infectious disease, substance abuse, and drug interactions or other risk factors that may influence the absorption, metabolism, distribution, or excretion of any medication prescribed.[1]

Physical and Mental Status Examination

Check for injury or intoxication including signs of toxic, infectious, or radioactive exposure. Pulse, blood pressure, and respiratory rate should be evaluated. New onset sustained hypertension or tachycardia is associated with later development of PTSD. Orientation, memory, mental content, anxiety, mood disturbance, or aggression must be addressed to rule out covert head injury. The Global Assessment of Functioning scale (GAF) is useful in estimating patients' ability to cope.[2]

Impact and Acute Phase: Goals of Psychopharmacology

The goals of acute post-disaster interventions include the following:

Assure safety
Reduce the symptom burden
Improve functioning

Psychopharmacological interventions in the context of acute disasters are usually prescribed on a short-term basis to reduce target symptoms, since they are not well studied.[3] Most uses of medication are off-label in acute disaster response since there are no FDA-approved indications specific to disaster. While this is true similarly for acute stress disorder, it is standard clinical practice to utilize anxiolytic, sedative, or antipsychotic medications for anxiety, insomnia, and agitation, in the same manner as when such interventions are clinically indicated for these presentations in primary care, emergency medicine, and consultation psychiatry (See Table 18.1 and Table 18.2).[4,5]

 Table 18.1 Impact Phase 0 to 48 hours: What to Expect

Feeling anxious, fearful, or stunned is normal and usually does not require patient intervention.

If patient is unable to organize himself or herself into accepting shelter, food, or assistance, or if intense anxiety prevents basic self-care, intervention is indicated.

A patient who is not eating, not drinking water, has palpitations, has shortness of breath, or has panic will benefit from intervention.

Patients who are agitated, paranoid, armed, or obsessed with a revenge attack require emergency intervention using ambulance or police services, if available.

Suicidal patients require a thorough psychiatric evaluation (see Chapter 7).

 Table 18.2 Acute Phase 48 hours to 2 months: What to Expect

Symptoms likely to present acutely:

Anxiety
Insomnia
Relapse of substance abuse (predominantly alcohol)

Symptoms less common but requiring urgent intervention:

Irritability with assaultiveness

Agitation when accompanied by intrusive thoughts, numbing, hypervigilance, irritability, verbal aggression, unable to sleep or rest.

Mania with elevated or irritable mood, grandiosity, pressured speech, no need for sleep, reckless spending, unusual promiscuity, intrusiveness, or altercations with security or police.

Anxiety

Among the most common presentations to primary care will be presentations of anxiety or somatic symptoms of anxiety, including palpitations, nausea, generalized weakness, or shortness of breath. After your brief medical work-up rules out disease and the possibility that the symptom(s) is part of a broader psychiatric disorder, consider treating the anxiety, with suggested interventions (see Table 18.3).

 Table 18.3 Pharmacological Interventions for Anxiety

Benzodiazepines

Anxiety, including panic symptoms, can be effectively reduced with low-dose benzodiazepines if given for a 7- or 14-day prescription.

Lorazepam 0.5 mg po qhs can be used bid or tid to a daily maximum of 4 mg for patients who are benzodiazepine naïve.

Clonazepam 0.5 mg po qhs or bid for 7 to 14 days only. Can be used bid or tid to a maximum of 4 mg per 24 hours.

Another benzodiazepine is diazepam.

Alternatives to Benzodiazepines

Buspirone 15 mg po bid or tid. A 1- or 2-week prescription sufficient until patient obtains psychiatric treatment.

Diphenhydramine (25–50 mg); this can be given qhs or bid for anxiety.

Hydroxyzine (10 mg, 25 mg, 50 mg); this can be given qhs or bid for anxiety.

Over-the-Counter Alternatives

Acetaminophen with diphenhydramine is an acceptable alternative for mild anxiety intervention.

Risks, Side Effects, and Drug Interactions

Sedation and dizziness are the most common side effects of benzodiazepines. In a very few individuals, disinhibited behavior can occur. Caution must be used in the elderly, in those with substance abuse issues, and in those with a history of dementia or delirium. Drug interactions for benzodiazepines include any drug with CNS sedation as a risk, including narcotics, mood stabilizers, or anti-seizure medications. Acetaminophen overdose may cause hepatic failure and death.

Benzodiazepine Dependence

After 21 days, there is evidence to suggest that the patient can become dependent and that withdrawal may occur with rebound insomnia and anxiety. Instruct the patient to use the medication for the first few nights, and then to taper if anxiety improves and use only on an as-needed basis. Caution must be used for benzodiazepines in the elderly who metabolize drugs slowly and in substance abusing patients. Generally speaking, psychopharmacological intervention for anxiety should include less than 1 week's worth of benzodiazepines to prevent tolerance and dependence.

Buspirone 15 mg po bid or tid was demonstrated in an open label study of 17 combat veterans to reduce re-experiencing symptoms on the PCL-C. This drug is FDA-approved for generalized anxiety. Buspirone has not been used for acute stress disorder, but might be effective for patients in whom a benzodiazepine is contraindicated.

Medication Strategies to Prevent PTSD

Propranolol is a beta blocker of interest in that it could block autonomic hyper-arousal and small case studies suggested benefit in preventing PTSD. Specifically, Pitman et al studied 41 emergency department patients within six hours of the event and randomized 18 patients to receive a 10-day course of double-blind propranolol 40 mg four times daily versus placebo. The results suggest that acute, post-trauma propranolol may have a preventive effect on subsequent PTSD.[6]

Insomnia

Insomnia is probably the most common presenting complaint after disaster. Your patients may report difficulty "turning off" their thoughts, and initial and middle insomnia are common.[7]

There are no trials of medication used for sleep disturbance in acute stress reactions, acute stress disorder, or PTSD, though these are widely used in an adjunctive fashion for their FDA-approved indication, which is short-term treatment of insomnia as shown in Table 18.4. Prescriptions for 14 days may be appropriate, after which time patients should seek a formal psychiatric consultation.[8]

Agitation

Though rare, agitation can be seen in the acute phase of disaster. Rumors of mass panic or group psychosis are just that: rumors. Agitated patients warrant a psychiatric referral for evaluation. Often there is an underlying mental illness, substance abuse, or other disorder; however, it is possible you may see agitation de novo in the acute stages of disaster, and possible pharmacological interventions to be considered are shown in Table 18.5.

Medical Work-up

For any patient presenting with agitation, a history must be obtained regarding recent alcohol or substance abuse, and appropriate urine or blood drug screens must be performed when possible. A CT scan or MRI is indicated in any patient with a history of head injury or trauma, or with complex underlying medical problems, such as cancer.

Mild Agitation with Extreme Anxiety

In patients for whom a benzodiazepine is contraindicated due to prior adverse reactions, very low doses of atypical anti-psychotics can be

 Table 18.4   Interventions for Insomnia

Zolpidem 10 mg po qhs or
Zolpidem CR 6.25 or 12.5 mg po qhs
Eszopiclone 1 or 2 mg po qhs

Ramelteon 8 mg po qhs

Trazodone 50 mg po qhs

Risks, Side Effects, and Drug Interactions

Sedation and dizziness are the most common side effects of medications for insomnia. In a very few individuals, disinhibited behavior can occur. Caution must be used in the elderly, in those with substance abuse issues, and in those with a history of dementia or delirium. Drug interactions for insomnia medication include any drug with CNS sedation as a risk, including benzodiazepines, narcotics, mood stabilizers, or anti-seizure medications.

Table 18.5   Interventions for Agitation

Agitation is managed in the same way as any acute ER presentation if the survivor is dangerous, extremely agitated, or psychotic. In the ER use:

Haloperidol 0.5–2 mg IM/po with
Lorazepam 1–2 mg IM/po
Diphenhydramine 50 mg IM/po can be given if there is concern for dystonic reactions.

Dose ranges for haloperidol: 0.5–2 mg po/ IM q4h prn for agitation
   Lorazepam 1–2 mg po/IM q4h prn for agitation
   Diphenhydramine 50 mg po/IM can also be given q4h

Risks, Side Effects, and Drug Interactions

Sedation and dizziness are the most common side effects of medications for agitation. Rarely, haloperidol can cause dystonic reactions in vulnerable patients. Young African American males, those with mood disorder histories, and the elderly require close monitoring for a dystonic reaction. Giving diphenhydramine in combination with haloperidol and Ativan is a precautionary measure against dystonic reactions.

Caution must be used in the elderly, where the doses can be used at the lowest range, and given less frequently. Benzodiazepines must be given with caution in elderly patients due to risk of falls and hip fractures or hypotension. Close monitoring and observation are important.

used to control agitation or extreme anxiety (See Table 18.6). All antipsychotic medications include warnings of dystonic reactions, neuroleptic malignant syndrome, or tardive dyskinesia. They also include a black box warning not to use them with patients who have dementia, due to risk of CVA including stroke, and there is increased risk of death in dementia-related psychosis. In patients taking atypical antipsychotics there is also risk of severe weight gain, hyperglycemia, and diabetes mellitus. In at-risk patients, an ECG is advised if possible. QTc prolongation is a risk of anti-psychotic and other medications and is associated with cardiac arrhythmia. Additionally, documentation should be provided clarifying why conventional approaches to agitation (including benzodiazepines or diphenhydramine) are not indicated or have been tried but have been ineffective. Two examples are low-dose risperidone and low-dose quetiapine.

Risperidone

0.5–1.0 mg po qhs or bid. Risperdone is a useful drug for refractory insomnia in PTSD when a benzodiazepine or other hypnotic is contraindicated or has failed. It is often an adjunct to an SSRI, rather than a replacement for the SSRI. In a recent study of 45 veterans receiving sertraline, risperidone augmentation produced gains in sleep and global assessment of functioning, though it did not decrease the overall rates of PTSD.[9]

Quetiapine

25–50 mg po qhs or bid. Quetiapine may be an appropriate agent to consider for off-label use, instead of a benzodiazepine, when the patient is anxious, agitated, with insomnia, and when a benzodiazepine has been either ineffective or is not appropriate. For example, in substance abusing patients during cocaine or amphetamine intoxication, or in patients who are on methadone where using a benzodiazepine risks respiratory depression, or in patients with prior brain injury, which is a relative contraindication for benzodiazepines.

Case Study: Agitation, threats of violence, probable chronic PTSD, possible alcohol withdrawal in an older man

After 9/11, Jim, an older man, comes in to the ER after working on the "bucket brigade" for 2 days. He complains that he feels angry and out of control and that he wants to kill the people who did this awful thing to his country. He was brought in by a friend who says he "went ballistic" at the food area when he saw an Asian man, yelling at him about Vietnam, and the destruction he had seen when he served there in the army 28 years ago. The patient has a gun at home, and he explains that his friend, who is also a Vietnam Veteran, lost a son in the attacks. He asks for a sedative to "just get calm." Here quetiapine 25 mg po may be a good choice, and a referral to psychiatry to assess his level of dangerousness is essential.

Post-Acute Phase Psychopharmacology

Sertraline is FDA-approved for post-traumatic stress disorder and major depression and can be started at lower doses and increased gradually.

Table 18.6 Post-Acute Phase 4 to 8 Weeks After Disaster

PTSD, Major Depression, and Substance Abuse

After the first 4 weeks, patients usually have managed to organize physical and emotional safety and support. Those who remain highly symptomatic with anxiety, insomnia, or numbing and detachment should be given a full screening interview for post-traumatic stress disorder, major depression, and substance abuse. If possible, this screening should include less typical disaster-associated problems such as generalized anxiety disorder and panic disorder.

Usually at this stage, an SSRI or other antidepressant (many of which have anti-anxiety indications or benefits) is indicated, while continuing as needed benzodiazepines or other medication for insomnia.

Ensure that the patient has follow-up with a psychiatrist after starting an antidepressant, as patients may not otherwise return for monitoring of treatment response or of adverse effects such as headache, diarrhea, or sexual side effects, which can affect adherence.

Commonly used SSRIs or SNRIs include sertraline, paroxetine, citalopram, fluoxetine, and venlafaxine.

For example, starting at 50 mg po qhs initially, and increasing to 150 mg as indicated. Side effects include dry mouth, headache, and sexual side effects.[10]

Paroxetine is FDA-approved for post-traumatic stress disorder and for major depression. Beginning with 10 mg po qhs, and titrating up to 20 mg po qhs, may be useful. Side effects are dry mouth, headache, sexual side effects, and weight gain.[11]

Citalopram prevented PTSD development in 15 acute burn victims while improving their wound healing.[12] Citalopram has also been used in open-label trials in small numbers of combat veterans with PTSD. Citalopram is generally used by psychiatrists when the patient is intolerant of sertraline or paroxetine.[13]

Venlafaxine has been studied in one randomized placebo controlled trial with 329 non-combat PTSD patients.[14] There are several open-label studies of venlafaxine for PTSD, and it is FDA-approved for generalized anxiety and panic disorder. Patients must be warned that if they discontinue medication abruptly, they may experience venlafaxine discontinuation syndrome. This includes headache, vertigo, and nausea.

Fluoxetine has been studied in 226 patients with PTSD, about half of them combat-related. At doses of 40 or 60 mg, after 6 weeks, the medication was superior to placebo, though incidence of treatment-emergent side effects was significant.[15]

Prazosin 0.5–10 mg po qhs, clonidine, and guanfacine have been studied in open-label trials in the combat veteran population for irritable aggression, hyper-arousal, and intrusive memories with some success. They are contraindicated in patients with cardiovascular disease, diabetes, or those who would be intolerant of a drop in blood pressure. The difficulty in titration and monitoring of these medications make them impractical in the acute disaster setting where dislocation of survivors makes follow-up unreliable. These medications are best used after first-line SSRIs and short-term low-dose benzodiazepines have failed.[8,16]

Substance Abuse Relapse

You should treat relapse in the same way as in usual primary care management, with psychiatric evaluation once detoxification has been completed.

Inpatient detoxification is indicated where available. In all cases emergency social services should provide patient with AA meetings and referral to outpatient substance abuse services.

Schizophrenia, Bipolar Disorder, and Other Severe and Persistent Mental Illness

Patients living in the community with schizophrenia or severe bipolar illness often lose their connection to mental health treatment temporarily or forget to refill their medication. Some become convinced that they must stay on guard and stop their anti-psychotic medications, believing that they may sleep through another disaster or terrorist attack, or believing that staying alert is imperative at all times. Patients with bipolar disorder may become activated, agitated, and develop sleep disturbance— a cardinal symptom of an impending manic episode, which may present with insomnia, pressured speech, irritability, elevated mood, or even assaultiveness.

Psychotropic Medication Maintenance

Discontinuation of psychotropic medications, either those started acutely postdisaster or previously, may in some patients result in increased symptoms of anxiety, depression, or psychosis. In developed countries, you are likely to play an essential role in providing refills for antipsychotic, antidepressant, or mood stabilizing medications. Some hospital psychiatry services can provide pharmaceutical samples or referral to psychiatric services. Directing the patient back to mental health care is very useful, or referring for hospital or day hospital admission if available and indicated.

Child and Adolescent Psychopharmacology in a Disaster

The general principles and standards of practice for child and adolescent psychiatry and for managing stress, insomnia, mood disturbances, agitation, and behavioral dyscontrol in pediatric medical settings may be relevant also in disasters. Collaboration with a child and adolescent psychiatrist or psychopharmacologist is ideal and is possible in disaster settings with telepsychiatry capability.[17,18] Dosing of medications for children differs from adults and is calculated according to pediatric dosing guidelines, on a milligram per kilogram basis.

Assessment

Pediatric Medical and Psychiatric History, Physical Exam, and Mental Status

Information gathered from the pediatric history, including the child psychiatric history and the physical and mental status examinations, guide psychopharmacological practice.

Particular attention should be paid to factors such as developmental immaturity, systemic illness, infectious disease, drug interactions, substance abuse, or other risk factors that may influence the absorption, metabolism, distribution, or elimination of any medication prescribed.

Assessment of very young children by primary care clinicians involves gaining knowledge of the maternal-infant and paternal-infant "dyad" in assessing the child's developmental status and response to the acute stress of disaster. Psychological interventions with the help of a caring, nurturing parent are often, but not always, remarkably calming to the stressed or agitated infant or young child. Psychological intervention can be even more calming than most medications, including reassurance, empathy, holding, and re-structuring the child's environment to guard against overstimulation and disruption of routine.

Diagnosis

Child psychiatric diagnoses such as PTSD or major depression in older children are similar to those for adults. Other conditions that might contribute to presenting symptoms include pediatric illness, injuries, infectious diseases, developmental disabilities, intellectual limitations, and learning disabilities and should be considered in the diagnostic assessment.

Treatment

As with adults, insomnia is a common manifestation of anxiety (although other causes need to be ruled out) in children under stress, including after disasters. Transient insomnia is unlikely to require medication, but persistent insomnia may benefit from the judicious therapeutic trial for 5 to 7 days of diphenhydramine, or if that is ineffective, of a benzodiazepine (or rarely of an atypical antipsychotic medication). If the insomnia is a symptom of PTSD, cognitive behavior therapy or an antidepressant may be more effective.

There is a limited base of evidence-informed research supporting sertraline, fluoxetine, and imipramine for ASD, PTSD, and depression in children.[18] There is an evidence base supporting fluoxetine for major depression.[19] Hyperactive children whose stimulant medication has been interrupted due to the disaster will likely benefit if it is resumed. Antidepressants in children and adolescents should optimally be used in collaboration with a child psychiatrist, as they carry an FDA black box warning for increased suicidal ideation, and as with adults, antidepressants may trigger a switch into a manic episode. However, with good follow-up care, psychotherapy, and close monitoring, treating childhood depression can be lifesaving. This may be particularly true for children who are injured, bereaved, or who experience other sudden losses in disaster.

Agitation in Children

Severe agitation in children is managed in collaboration with a pediatrician or child and adolescent psychiatrist. Increasingly, in developed countries, atypical antipsychotics, such as risperidone, quetiapine, olanzapine (available in dissolving form), and aripiprazole may be used off-label for severe agitation with dosing by weight. For 2- to 6-year-old children, diphenhydramine and/or a benzodiazepine may be effective and are widely used, again with dosing by weight.[18]

All medications, except in older adolescents, are dosed according to the weight of the child. For anxiety, short-acting benzodiazepines are usually safe anxiolytic agents. Unless there is a past history of disinhibition, concerns about disinhibition generally do not preclude the use of these agents if the child is supervised by a responsible parent or guardian; the medication should be stopped if disinhibition occurs. High doses or slowed metabolic excretion carry the risk of respiratory depression.

Conclusion

In considering psychopharmacological treatment after disaster, your history and physical examination should focus on both pre-existing as well as disaster-related factors that may influence your patient's response to a medication. Typically treatment is directed toward symptoms of distress and common disorders after traumatic experience such as anxiety or panic, insomnia, depression, or agitation. The goal is to manage symptoms and to develop treatment relationships with patients such that they can access follow-up psychopharmacologic care in the post-acute disaster phase should symptoms persist or become syndromes. Important considerations during disaster are relapse or new onset of substance abuse or withdrawal, which are managed in the same way that they usually are in primary care. Be alert for elderly, impoverished, or severely mentally ill patients who have discontinued their prescribed medications and have developed symptoms as a result. Patient safety is paramount.

- Use common sense.
- Prescribe the lowest effective dosages.
- Encourage the patient to take the medication for the duration prescribed.
- Ensure that there is a follow-up appointment in the community.
- Follow-up should address any adverse effects, assure that the medication and dosage selected are correct and beneficial, and, if necessary, should provide refills or a different medication.

References

1. Alpert JE, Fava M, Rosenbaum JF. Psychopharmacologic issues in the medical setting. In: Stern TA, Fricchione GL, Cassem NH, Jellinek MS, Rosenbaum JF, Eds. *Massachusetts General Hospital Handbook of General Hospital Psychiatry*. 5th ed. Philadelphia, PA: Mosby/Elsevier; 2004:231–268.

2. American Psychiatric Association. *Diagnostic and Statistical Manual of Mental Disorders, Fourth Edition, Text Revision*. Arlington, VA: American Psychiatric Association Publishers; 2000.

3. Friedman M. The role of pharmacotherapy in early interventions. In: Blumenfield M, Ursano RJ, Eds. *Interventions and Resilience After Mass Trauma*. Cambridge: Cambridge University Press; 2008.

4. Katz C. Early Therapeutic Interventions Post-Disaster: Psychopharmacology. March 27, 2008, presentation at the New York City chapter of Voluntary Organizations Active in Disaster (VOAD), New York, NY.

5. Stoddard FJ, Levine JB, Lund K. Burn injuries. In: Blumenfield M, Strain J, Eds. *Psychosomatic Medicine*. Philadelphia, PA: Lippincott Williams & Wilkins; 2006:309–336.

6. Pitman RK, Sanders KM, Zusman RM, Healy AR, Cheema F, Lasko, et al. Pilot study of secondary prevention of post-traumatic stress disorder with propranolol. *Biological Psychiatry*. 2002;51(2):189–192.

7. Mellman TA, Pigeon WR, Nowell PD, Nolan B. Relationships between REM sleep findings and PTSD symptoms during the early aftermath of trauma. *J Trauma Stress*. 2007;20(5):893–901.

8. National Center for PTSD. Pharmacological Treatment of Acute Stress Reactions and PTSD: A Fact Sheet for Providers. 2008. Available at: **http://www.ncptsd.va.gov**. Accessed March 31, 2008.

9. Rothbaum BO, Killeen TK, Davidson JR, Brady KT, Connor KM, Heekin MH. Placebo-controlled trial of risperidone augmentation for selective serotonin reuptake inhibitor-resistant civilian post-traumatic stress disorder. *J Clin Psychiatry*. 2008;69(4):520–525.

10. Friedman M, et al. Randomized, double-blind comparison of sertraline and placebo for post-traumatic stress disorder in a Department of Veterans Affairs setting. *J Clin Psychiatry*. 2007;68(5):711–720.

11. Stein DJ, et al. Paroxetine in the treatment of post-traumatic stress disorder: pooled analysis of placebo-controlled studies. *Expert Opin Pharmacother*. 2003;4(10):1829–1838.

12. Bláha J, et al. Therapeutical aspects of using citalopram in burns. *Acta Chir Plast*. 1999;41(1):25–32.

13. English BA, et al. Treatment of chronic post-traumatic stress disorder in combat veterans with citalopram: an open trial. *J Clin Psychopharmacol.* 2006;26(1):84–88.

14. Davidson J, et al. Treatment of post-traumatic stress disorder with venlafaxine extended release: a 6-month randomized controlled trial. *Arch Gen Psychiatry.* 2006;63(10):1158–1165.

15. Martenyi F, et al. Fluoxetine versus placebo in post-traumatic stress disorder. *J Clin Psychiatry.* 2002;63(3):199–206.

16. Miller LJ. Prazosin for the treatment of post-traumatic stress disorder sleep disturbances. *Pharmacotherapy.* 2008;28(5):656–666.

17. Martin A, Scahill L, Charney DS, Leckman JF, eds. *Pediatric Psychopharmacology: Principles and Practice.* New York, NY: Oxford University Press; 2003.

18. Stoddard F, Usher C, Abrams A. Psychopharmacology in pediatric critical care: child adolescent psychiatric. *Clin N Am.* 2006;(15):611–655.

19. Tsapakis EM, Soldani F, Tondo L, Baldessarini RJ. Efficacy of antidepressants in juvenile depression: meta-analysis. *Br J Psychiatry.* 2008;193(1):10–17.

Collaborative Care

Todd F. Holzman, MD

Peter, working in medical triage, waves to the collaborating psychiatrist, for an urgent consult. A man in his mid-20s evacuated from the Katrina disaster is agitated, not making sense, and seems very odd. He reveals he has been hearing frightening, commanding voices for several years, sleeping very poorly, and barely managing, living on the margins of society. Alcohol had made the voices worse, so he no longer drinks. He has not had any medical or psychiatric help in the past but would very much like to be rid of the voices. After being medically cleared, available haloperidol was begun and referral to state mental health clinic initiated. His improvement in the structured shelter environment was dramatic over the next week. The voices greatly diminished, he felt emotionally relieved, and he participated in limited, structured, and communal chores with satisfaction and social acceptance. Extensive and invaluable collaboration included work not only between Peter and his collaborating psychiatrist, but also with professionals in substance abuse, shelter security, housing and kitchen facilities, and state mental health and rehabilitation services.

- Today's medical care is collaborative team care. Easy accessibility of mental health clinicians is essential after disasters.
- When? Collaboration occurs at all phases of disasters, by telepsychiatry if necessary.
- What for? Collaborative care assists primary care clinicians in assessment, management, and in planning aftercare.
- Examples include suicidality, MUPS, psychosis, substance abuse, injured patients, and community outreach.
- How do you collaborate effectively? This is done by getting to know your mental health colleagues over time, clearly framing questions, and what you need.
- What about follow-up? Sharing feedback on what worked and what didn't helps as does working to further enhance your collaborative teamwork to improve care.

Collaborative Care

Today's medical care is increasingly team care, and this is even truer in health care after disasters. It is of great interest that "many generalist physicians provide an historical example of shared care transforming inter-professional relations."[1] With clinicians much more aware of the mental health needs of their patients and too few mental health professionals available, primary care clinicians including doctors, nurses, and others increasingly provide mental health care collaboratively with psychiatrists, psychologists, clinical social workers, and substance abuse counselors. In disasters, this model is even more needed. Collaborative mental health care after disasters is a central part of optimal care and effective medical teamwork.

Accessibility and Identification of Mental Health Clinicians

Collaborative care can benefit your contacts with disaster responders, especially security, fire and rescue, and other public services. It is an essential element of disaster planning and best integrated into each phase of effective preparedness, including preparing together with mental health professionals as part of the team. This may increase the likelihood of having them on-site, rather than working from a distance or not part of the disaster team.

New models for collaborative care are rapidly emerging. They are being elaborated in primary care generally, and in collaboration with nursing, including measures to evaluate the effectiveness of communication and collaboration.[1–3] Models, such as the Massachusetts Child Psychiatry Access Project (MCPAP), are being adopted in several states for rapid phone and email contact between psychiatrists and child psychiatrists with primary care clinicians and pediatricians who prescribe the bulk of psychotropic medications.[4] For traumatized children, Saxe et al have developed a collaborative care model called Trauma Systems Therapy to assess mental health problems in children and their families, identify the problems and the service systems involved, initiate treatment, and improve patient outcomes.[5] This is trauma-focused, and, whether in the community or in a health care facility, brings together the relevant health professionals, especially primary care clinicians and mental health professionals, around particular cases of traumatized children to evaluate and identify/diagnose the problems in the system, including home, school, health care and other agencies, the barriers to effective outcomes, recommended solutions and treatments, those who are the providers, and evaluation of the results. This has been used with victims of sexual trauma, refugees, and other child trauma victims. A different but related approach called Preschool Trauma Therapy (PTT) has been developed to reduce stress in both traumatized preschoolers and in their parents.[6] With adults, in a different but similar collaborative care model, Zatzick et al found that injured patients prioritize their needs differently from clinicians, which then informs clinicians how to focus interventions more effectively, improving outcomes.[7,8] Such models could have a place in disaster response in order to improve the delivery of mental health care.

While there is often concern about the stigma of having contact with mental health clinicians, easy identification of these clinicians reduces stigma and allows for immediate contact during a crisis when survivors need to find help with little confusion or delay. Obvious identification, such as a colored dot on clinicians' name tags, same color baseball caps, or vests might be appropriate. Phone, location, and other mental health professional contact information facilitate medical, security, clergy, and all other responders making the most rapid consultation response possible. On-call clinicians with rapid contact information should be easily accessible.

Allocation of Space for Collaboration

The organization of locations and accessibility for mental health and substance abuse clinicians should follow survivor flow. Mental health presence is helpful at reception areas for greeting, orientation, and triage. Screening areas are best arranged with easy access to and from medical/surgical areas. Adequate clinical mental heath consultation and treatment space should be designated and private. Primary care benefits from mental health contact in common areas for survivors and families, where they can eat, talk, and receive news, and appropriate and distinct areas for children and adolescents should be arranged. Mental health presence at security checkpoints and with the medical examiner and mortuary services is optimal. Casual behavioral health contact to allow survivors to "tell their stories" at any desired time to a compassionate, receptive listener may reduce the burden of patients seeking primary care services.

Meeting the Needs of Family and Friends

Communication and reunification with family, friends, and other individuals close to survivors are of great importance. Identification and tracking systems, with whatever electronic or personal communications are available, require sufficient space and facilities for many additional people. All these individuals will want information about their survivor's condition, medical treatment, prognosis, as well as direct personal contact. Casual, informal mental health collaboration can be very useful in these circumstances and can help lower anxiety levels. Also, family or friends may be shocked by the realization there may be only partial or no remains available when they arrive at the medical examiner area or mortuary seeking information. This is another critical area for mental health collaborative support.

Evaluation

It is useful to evaluate the quality of primary care mental health collaboration in order to try to further improve communication and patient care. Evaluation surveys (e.g., Press Ganey) are administered to patients and families, other team members, primary care clinicians, and mental health professionals to rate the quality of services. This is currently done in many health care facilities and might be extended to monitor satisfaction and quality in disaster health care.

References

1. Stoeckle JD, Ronan LJ, Emmanuel L, Ehrlich C, Hughes CC. *Doctoring Together: A Physician's Guide to Manners, Duties, and Communication in the Shared Care of Patients.* Boston, MA: Massachusetts General Hospital Primary Care Division; 2002:13.

2. LaValley D. Physician-nurse collaboration and patient safety. *The Forum.* 2008;26(2).

3. Fewster-Thuente L, Velsor-Friedrich B. Interdisciplinary collaboration for health care professionals. *Nurs Adm Q.* 2008;32(1):409–448.

4. Massachusetts Child Psychiatry Access Project (MCPAP). Available at **http://mcpap.typepad.com/**. Accessed March 3, 2009.

5. Saxe GN, Ellis BH, Kaplow J. *Collaborative Treatment of Traumatized Children and Teens: The Trauma Systems Therapy Approach.* New York, NY: Guilford; 2006.

6. Stoddard FJ, Murphy JM, Chedekel DS, Sorrentino E, Saxe GN, White G. A Randomized Controlled Trial of Preschool Trauma Therapy (PTT), (Manuscript in preparation). March 2009.

7. Zatzick D. Collaborative care for injured victims of individual and mass trauma: a health services research approach to developing early interventions. In: Ursano RJ, Fullerton CS, Norwood AE, Eds. *Terrorism and Disaster: Individual and Community Mental Health Interventions.* Cambridge: Cambridge University Press; 2003:189–205.

8. Zatzick DF, Russo J, Rajotte E, Uehara E, Roy-Byrne P, Ghesquiere A, et al. Strengthening the patient-provider relationship in the aftermath of physical trauma through an understanding of the nature and severity of post-traumatic concerns. *Psychiatry.* 2007;70(3):260–273.

Staff Support

Joseph P. Merlino, MD, MPA

Dr. Jonathan Fox was the medical director of a large primary care clinic located in a town that experienced a bridge collapse with mass casualties. While no clinic staff members died in the collapse, employees had relatives or friends who perished in the disaster. No one it seemed was unaffected. The collapse occurred during the Friday morning rush-hour commute. Dr. Fox decided to close the clinic at noon that day since many staff could not get to the office and those who did arrive wanted to be home with family members. A notice was put on the clinic's front door, web page, and phone answering service directing patients in need of care to the local hospital. Dr. Fox remained at his desk thinking about what the next week would bring for his clinic and its staff.

That weekend he decided to call a good friend of his who was an expert in human resources. He also called the shop steward of the union, to which many of his staff belonged, and a member of his senior medical staff to coordinate and plan how to proceed. Everyone agreed that for the next several days, it wouldn't be "business as

- Take the time and resources *now* to plan how you and your organization would respond in the event of a disaster. Each workplace is different, and your needs may be unique. One of many resources to help you plan is that of the American Red Cross, which features a section on Preparing and Getting Trained, available online at: http://www.red cross.org.

- Involve staff from all areas of your organization in putting your specific plan together.

- Once a policy and procedure has been formalized, be sure everyone is regularly educated and trained.

- Review your document periodically and update it accordingly.

usual." Everyone also agreed how much they wished they'd put together a disaster preparedness policy earlier that they could refer to now.

The shop steward told Dr. Fox that she had a telephone tree that was used in previous "get out the vote" events. They decided to activate this to see which employees could come to work Monday and which staff needed assistance and would not be able to report. Those needing assistance would be followed-up by a clinic representative and referred to appropriate clinic and community support services (e.g., financial, medical, psychological). Appropriate HR policies would be activated ensuring covered time off, salary, benefits, and so forth. The clinics contacting staff would be reassuring and comforting to affected staff, demonstrating the caring of the organization and the concern for its clinical staff and other employees. Jonathan made sure that HR would continue to follow these individuals as long as necessary or appropriate.

Planning next proceeded to what to do on Monday morning. It was agreed to have a general staff meeting for those able to report to share and update information and to focus immediately on the issues listed in Box 20.1.

Box 20.1   Planning

- Emotional support for each member of the staff
- Information sharing
  - Those staff not at work were contacted and were assisted as needed
  - Acknowledgment of what occurred and that it had affected everyone
  - Assurance that information sharing would be ongoing
  - Staff support would be ongoing as long as needed and appropriate
  - Individual needs would be addressed individually and confidentially as required
  - Work assignments and changes required to keep the clinic functioning as optimally as possible would occur including shortened open hours if necessary so that staff:
    - Could attend memorial services and funerals
    - Volunteer in the field as needed

Dr. Fox was himself reassured by the fact that he now had something of a plan for how to proceed. He knew that if he could get through Monday morning, he and others could plan effectively for the days ahead. Wisely, the shop steward made sure that *all* staff was included in the telephone calls and staff meetings; this included housekeepers, security guards, cafeteria staff, as well as front office and management. This had the effect of bringing all the staff emotionally closer together and assisted in those needing extra help and support being identified by confidantes who otherwise would not have been included in organizational meetings.

During the Monday morning staff meeting, Dr. Fox asked if a group could get together at the end of the day to reflect on what had happened and how it was impacting some of the staff. A voluntary meeting of interested persons was set up. One of the clinic's nurses contacted a nearby mental health center to request that one of their staff facilitate the meeting. So many staff showed up that it was necessary to run two separate groups every few days for the remainder of the week. In addition to the obvious issues that came up for discussion, the processing of the sensitive and important matter of staff-staff friction and staff-leadership friction was key to the ongoing smooth operation of the clinic. During disasters emotions run high and when the anger "at the disaster" can't be pinned on someone or something, colleagues and leadership often are targeted instead. The skillful facilitation of the group meetings enabled the emotions to flow but also provided for the constructive channeling of these emotions and the provision of explanations about friction in such situations so that the staff could move beyond their anger and more appropriately deal with their grief, fear, and frustration. Gradually, staff rebounded and only one group was required twice a week and then once a week thereafter for the next few months.

Soon thereafter, the staff who were not able to report to work at the clinic that first Monday returned and were welcomed and integrated back into a caring and supportive environment that seemingly grew stronger through the adversity they shared.

A few weeks later, Dr. Fox convened a task force of all levels of staff to assess their clinic's response, noting what worked well and what actions made clear the need for changes in policy and readiness. After the review was completed, an updated disaster preparedness plan was formalized for the clinic, disseminated widely, and staff training begun.

In putting together their plan, Dr. Fox and his colleagues utilized an excellent document from the Federal Emergency Management Agency (FEMA), entitled *Emergency Management Guide for Business and Industry*, which is available online at **http://www.fema.gov/pdf/business/ guide/bizindst.pdf.**

This guide emphasizes that since employees who will rely on you for support after an emergency are your most valuable asset, you need to consider the range of services that you could provide or arrange for, including those listed in Box 20.2.

In addition to the direct delivery of care, health practitioners can also offer invaluable support, guidance, and advice to the administrators and managers of other facilities and organizations pertaining to their overall preparedness and response (see Box 20.3).

An example of this occurred during the 9/11 atrocities in New York City. Mental health staff from neighboring New York University Med-

Box 20.2 Emergency Management Guide

- Cash advances
- Salary continuation
- Flexible work hours
- Reduced work hours
- Crisis counseling
- Care packages
- Day care

Box 20.3 Helping Others Prepare

Helping can take various forms, including:
- Assisting other facilities to develop care plans in the event of a future disaster
- Offering direction during events in order to maximize positive outcomes and minimize negative outcomes

ical Center-Bellevue Hospital Center assisted the leadership of the Office of the Chief Medical Examiner (the city morgue) in the editing of pamphlets being prepared for families who lost someone in the 9/11 attacks. The sensitivity of the mental health staff was crucial in selecting the appropriate tone that the scientists of the OCME wished to convey to those grieving and acutely dealing with the effects of disaster and loss.

Collaborations like the examples in this chapter have the potential for strengthening the linkages necessary for a community's recovery while also giving individuals a sense of purpose so important for the support of staff during times of crisis and disaster response.

International Disaster Perspectives: Issues and Challenges

Anthony T. Ng, MD

When Peter heard about the Asian tsunamis, he was saddened and was very upset as he had worked in Sri Lanka as a medical student during his training. Additionally, he is an internist working in a diverse community in Boston that includes South Asians and many other immigrant groups. There is also a university campus in the community that has a large number of overseas exchange students. Peter was wondering how he can be of help given his past connections to the affected area. He felt his professional skills and clinical experiences could be useful. However, he noticed that many of his patients were equally if not more upset and distressed by the disaster. Many of them were concerned about their families and friends back home, and many expressed frustrations due to the lack of information and wanted to know how they could be of help. Peter is feeling somewhat frustrated as to how he can best help his patients and also as to how he can help the people directly affected in South Asia.

- All large disasters have global impacts on mental health.

- Survivors of disasters have unique mental health considerations and needs in the international setting.

- Ethnic and expatriate communities are at high risk of experiencing stigma, victimization, and mental health distress from disasters overseas.

- A public health and community focus is essential to strengthen resiliency in international disasters.

- Primary care clinicians have opportunities to make significant contributions to the mental and emotional well-being of those affected even when disaster occurs overseas.

Introduction

The impacts of disasters internationally have been severe in most instances. In the past decades, there have been several major disasters that have caused substantial damage and destruction and have led to major public health responses. These included the 9/11 terrorist attacks, the Asian tsunamis in 2004, Hurricane Katrina, and the more recent cyclone in Myanmar and earthquake in China. The tremendous psychiatric consequences on the affected populations have been documented in many of these events. Overall, with increasing connections between communities worldwide, disasters anywhere have impacts in distant communities. It is important for primary care clinicians like Peter to increase their awareness and understanding of the nature of international disasters, as well as the psychiatric consequences that result when these events occur, and how they can help their patients and communities.

Nature of International Disasters

International disasters have special characteristics that can influence their scale and impact. It is helpful to consider international disasters from two domains—nature of the event and characteristics of the foreign communities impacted by them. It is important to differentiate the types of disasters seen in industrialized nations in the world, which may be very similar to what may occur in the United States. These may include natural disasters, such as earthquakes and storms. There may also be severe drought resulting in famine and population displacement. Disasters may also be man-made, such as aviation or industrial disasters, as well as acts of terrorism. Additional man-made disasters can also include industrial accidents, such as the toxic gas accident in Bhopal, India, or more commonly conflicts, such as war and civil strife, as in Rwanda and Sudan. In non-industrialized regions of the world such as Myanmar or Sri Lanka, disasters tend to be more severe and widespread. Perhaps the *major differences between international and domestic disasters* are that international disasters involve massive public health consequences, including mental health consequences, and that they kill, injure, and cause terrible emotional suffering to tens of thousands of people (or more) living in densely populated areas.[1] And another critical difference is that the poorest countries lack the infrastructure and resources (disaster services, food, shelter, health care) to respond to the tragedy.

In appreciating the impacts of international disasters, it is important that one appreciates the communities in which such events occur. In general, the more advanced infrastructure of industrialized nations limits the extent of the effects of disasters, mental health or otherwise. However, disasters in developing regions of the world, such as Africa, Asia, and South America, usually result in terrible mental health consequences from the greater damage to property and loss of life and greater likelihood of displaced persons and refugees. Non-industrialized nations tend to be most vulnerable. There are often more people living per square mile than in industrialized nations, with fewer resources. The housing and public infrastructure tends to be poorly built compared to developed countries, as was seen after the recent earthquake in China with its devastating school damage and loss of lives due to poor construction standards. Health and mental health infrastructures similarly tend to be less mature and stable prior to disasters. Additionally, there may be existing civil, ethnic, and political strife as in Sri Lanka and in Israel, Lebanon, the West Bank and Gaza. Last, emergency management planning and mental health are often not priorities for many struggling non-industrialized nations.

International Disasters and the United States

As international disasters often overwhelm local and regional resources quickly, the international community is more and more being called upon to assist. The United States in particular plays significant roles in disaster responses, such as to the Asian tsunamis and earthquakes in India, by providing logistics, material and personnel resources, as well as funding and technical assistance.[2] Such relief support can be from both civilian and military agencies of the U.S. federal government as well as the World Health Organization and from transnational non-governmental organizations (NGOs).

While the focus of the world may be on communities directly affected in international disasters, clinicians in the United States need be aware and to appreciate their global impacts. The United States is becoming increasingly diverse with many immigrants, both recent ones as well as others with longstanding family ties overseas. Others may be green card holders or expatriates such as workers and students residing in the United States. There are also communities with many undocumented aliens. Many of these individuals reside in the many ethnic communities located throughout the United States, especially in large urban areas. When disaster occurs overseas, members of the affected communities also experience disaster stress—but from a distance. They may be equally traumatized by disaster and its aftermath. Unlike their counterparts in the affected country, they are not dealing with the immediate needs of a post-disaster environment such as food, water, and shelter to distract them from experiencing anxiety, guilt, and grief about the impact of a disaster on their families overseas in the disaster region. Expatriate communities in the United States may have worries about their families and friends back home. Information about their well-being, as well as the status of the disaster response, will likely be scarce. Any information will likely be through the media and government sources. Many expatriates and immigrants experience anger and sadness, as well as frustration and helplessness at not being able to do more for the home communities. Their needs may be overshadowed by those of the affected overseas communities. Many immigrant populations may already have a high level of pre-existing psychiatric issues and past trauma. Thus, immigrant communities are often at great risk of developing adverse psychiatric conditions as a result of *indirect* exposure to disaster.[3]

Mental Health Roles and Opportunities in Primary Care

While overseas disasters do not have direct physical impact on the communities in the United States, indirect effects are often widespread and primary care clinicians have important roles here due to indirect trauma exposure. Most important, primary care clinicians can address the needs of those who have been traumatized or aggrieved by the disaster overseas due to their connections with friends and family in affected countries. Many individuals may suffer secondary traumatization from media coverage such as TV news and Internet. There may be others for whom media exposure may retrigger or exacerbate pre-existing psychiatric conditions, including PTSD as a result of indirect secondary trauma. Clinicians can monitor psychiatric sequelae and provide support for distressed individuals. As with any disaster survivors, it is important not to force them to relive their trauma experiences, to listen without judgment, and not to label them with psychiatric diagnoses, including post-traumatic stress disorder when screening for mental health issues (see Chapter 8).[4] In the example of Peter, he has an important and effective role in identifying and addressing the psychiatric needs of his patients who are experiencing psychiatric distress from their direct and indirect connections to the Asian tsunamis. He can identify and address needs both alone as well as in collaboration with another mental health provider (see Chapter 19).

For many in immigrant communities, psychiatric distress may present as somatic complaints. As a primary care clinician, you can provide psychiatric education to the community about distress, anxiety, and somatic complaints. Such information may not only benefit those in the communities here in the United States, but also this information may later be shared by members of the community with their families and friends overseas. Clinicians can promote, facilitate, and engage in outreach to educate communities about how they can address psychiatric concerns, including how best to care for those who are mentally ill. Such efforts are best done in collaboration with community leaders who may serve as brokers especially for immigrant communities that may experience mental health problems as stigmatizing. Other areas of outreach may include the workplace, places of worship, schools, and universities.

For clinicians interested in contributing their time and expertise to the medical response efforts overseas, they will need to be aware of the system of response such as which NGOs provide disaster response.[5] Such organizations can help facilitate credentialing, logistics, and deployment issues for staff and volunteers, including health providers. Prior to going overseas, clinicians should be aware of the environment they will encounter in the disaster zone, including the numbers of injuries and deaths, disruptions to families, extent of damage, potential for violence, ongoing or emerging public health concerns, and levels of political and civil strife. Basic needs and public sanitation may constitute risks for clinicians. Clinicians should be aware of language and cultural issues that may be present. Some knowledge of the past history of the affected region is helpful, including what the local perceptions are to outside or Western help. It is optimal for clinicians to learn about the organizational structure of disaster response and potential organizations that they can collaborate with in the region they are serving.

When deployed overseas, the first mental health intervention is planning and performing self-care for oneself, the primary care clinician, and planning how best to cope with the known and unknown stresses of time, distance from home, culture, and the context of the disaster (see Chapters 3 and 4). Major differences between international interventions and those in the United States are cultural, linguistic, and political mental health challenges as well as the probable enormous scale of suffering of the people affected. It is especially important to emphasize just how much that the suffering individuals, families, and communities benefit from the services of primary care clinicians who volunteer to serve overseas in organized disaster relief efforts.[6]

Conclusion

Disasters are increasingly complex and have wide and extended implications for communities globally.[7] Whether a disaster occurs here or overseas, communities here are affected, and primary care clinicians are at the forefront of identifying and responding to the mental health needs of those affected. You should be aware of faraway disasters as they may influence and impact the mental health of your patients and their communities. Your direct and collaborative mental health interventions in your own community have benefit for the health and well-being of those here and far beyond these shores.

References

1. Toole MJ, Waldman RJ. The public health aspects of complex emergencies and refugee situations. *Ann Rev Public Health.* 1997;18:283–312.

2. Tarantino D. Asian tsunami relief: Department of Defense public health response: policy and strategic coordination considerations. *Mil Med.* 2006;171(10):15–18.

3. Ng A. Cultural diversity in the integration of disaster mental health and public health: a case study in response to bioterrorism. *Int J Emerg Ment Health.* 2005;7:23–31.

4. Freedy JR, Simpson WM, Jr. Disaster-related physical and mental health: a role for the family physician. *Am Fam Physician.* 2007;75:841–846.

5. Sexana S, van Ommeren M, Saraceno B. Mental health assistance to populations affected by disasters: World Health Organization's role. *Int Rev Psych.* 2006;18:199–204.

6. Patel V, Garrison P, Mari JJ, Minas H, Prince M, Saxena S, and on behalf of the advisory group of the Movement for Global Mental Health. The Lancet's Series on Global Mental Health: 1 year on. *Lancet.* 2008, October 11;372(9646):1354–1357.

7. Merson M, Black R, Mills A. *International Public Health: Diseases, Programs, Systems, and Policies.* Sudbury, MA: Jones and Bartlett Publishers; 2005.

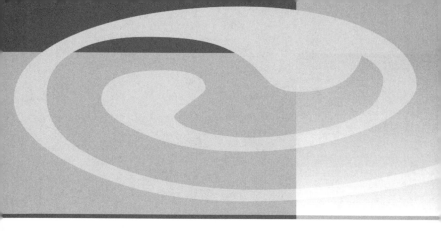

4

Special Issues

Section Editor: Frederick J. Stoddard Jr, MD

Use of Telepsychiatry: Implications in Disaster

Anthony T. Ng, MD

You are the sole primary care clinician in a small community in western Nebraska. Your community recently experienced a mass shooting at the local mall. In the 1 month since the shooting, many of your patients have been presenting with various unexplained somatic concerns, as well as many others who are reporting a varying range of mental health issues, including depression, anxiety, and signs and symptoms suggestive of post-traumatic stress disorder. Prior to the disaster, you would refer any individual with psychiatric symptoms to the community mental health clinic, which is an hour away and usually has an almost two-week long waiting list. However, due to the recent increased demand for mental health services, you decided to contact the university and see if it can assist you in another way. Since you had been using videoconferencing for some medical consults from your clinic, the university recommended that if individuals choose, they can receive a psychiatric consultation via videoconferencing and then the psychiatric consultant will make recommendations for initial mental health treatment, including psychiatric medication that you can initiate,

- As resources are quickly overwhelmed in disaster, telepsychiatry can be a viable option to access quality mental health support for health care providers in disaster.
- Limitations in the clinical use of telepsychiatry include dependence on audiovisual contact and the continued existence of infrastructure support (e.g., electricity, phone lines) as well as little evidence to support its use in disasters.
- Primary care clinicians need to be aware of ethical and legal regulations, if applicable, surrounding the use of telepsychiatry through their state professional licensing organizations and boards.
- The development and implementation of telepsychiatry will need to occur at the levels of the individual clinician, health care organization, and public health system.

until the patient is connected to a clinic. Additionally, you can also access via email and telephone several psychiatrists who have experience in trauma for more informal consultations.

Introduction

One of the most challenging aspects of providing care of any type in disasters and other mass public health emergencies is the scarcity of resources. This scarcity may be due to pre-existing conditions in the affected communities as well as due to the scale and severity of the disasters. Psychiatric and other mental health services also face such challenges. Prior to disasters, many communities have insufficient funding and resources to address the mental heath needs of their populations, resulting in long wait times for patients to be evaluated as well as lengthy delays in follow-up appointments. This causes delay in provision of, or failure to provide, critical psychiatric services. Patients often cannot obtain psychiatric help until their symptoms have become severe and impairing. This lack of psychiatric resources to prevent illness or provide early treatment for those with psychiatric problems becomes even more pronounced in times of disasters. Primary care clinicians, who are already providing such a broad range of medical services, can be central to efforts to address these mental health needs during and following disasters.

Evolving Training, Technologies, and Content

There has been great focus on developing trained mental health professionals who can respond to disasters and public health emergencies. Training of psychiatrists, psychologists, social workers, nurses, and other clinicians in disaster mental health is important as part of disaster planning and response. The development of, and investment in, telepsychiatry or telebehavioral health, which includes child and adolescent psychiatry, substance abuse, and other psychiatric subspecialties, can be an important complement to such planning and response. Telepsychiatry may occur via several different modes of communication, which continue to evolve.

A psychiatric consultant may be accessed via direct videoconferencing —during which a patient is evaluated—through an Internet connection.

It can also be done via telephone, PDA, or email if videoconferencing capability is unavailable.[1,2] The consultation may be for direct patient evaluation or consultation in how to address particular clinical concerns, especially from trauma and disaster experts in the case of telepsychiatry in disaster situations. Telepsychiatry, as a tool, is also increasingly used to evaluate and treat individuals with psychiatric emergencies.[3,4] Last, telepsychiatry-based continuing education courses for clinicians are expanding rapidly via the Internet and web sites, teaching about a full range of psychiatric issues, such as disaster psychiatry, cross-cultural mental health, child psychiatry, assessment, treatment of disorders such as PTSD and depression, and special topics in psychopharmacology.

Benefits

Numerous studies have demonstrated the efficacy and cost effectiveness of telemedicine, especially in the area of telepsychiatry, for assessment, treatment, and consultation.[5,6] Some studies have found that telepsychiatry, in which patients were assessed via video, is as reliable as in-person assessments.[7,8] This has been demonstrated with depression, anxiety disorders, and PTSD.[9,10] Regarding the use of telepsychiatry in treatment, one study showed there was no significant differences in outcomes between two groups of patients with combat-related PTSD, one in the same room and the other via telepsychiatry, who were given 14 weekly, 90-minute cognitive-behavioral therapy (CBT) treatment sessions.[10] "Strong" satisfaction was indicated by both groups. Other studies find equal satisfaction by both patients and providers in the use of telemedicine in treatment.[11,12] Telemedicine has also been used extensively for many years in military medicine, especially by the U.S. Navy to provide shipboard medical care far at sea, although it likely began with the invention of the telegraph and telephone. It is now in widespread use in all branches of the military and has been demonstrated to help in consultation roles in disasters as well as assessments of patients.[13–15]

In disaster situations, various issues may trigger need for psychiatric consultation. Telepsychiatry may offer one type of solution to the lack of psychiatric expertise (and other medical resources) as a result of the surge of mental health issues that arise after a disaster, acutely and over the long term. Psychiatric resources may be able to be used without the need to transport patients over long distances. This can help minimize risks to clinicians by negating the need to expose them to the risks of the disaster scene. An example would be in the event of a pandemic outbreak where mobility is restricted and the population, including psychiatric clinicians, may be quarantined.

Limitations

As telepsychiatry is innovative and potentially useful in a disaster, its use is still full of challenges due to not being with the patient, legal and ethical issues, access to the IT infrastructure, and "administrative buy-in." Telepsychiatry may not offer the benefit of direct interpersonal interactions that are often much needed by patients after a disaster. In addition, there needs to be an infrastructure, such as some type of pre-existing telecommunication networks, available for its use. Even if such infrastructure is in place, some disasters are so disruptive that the basic infrastructure of communications and utilities is destroyed or compromised. Staff may not be adequately trained in its use and those who are knowledgeable may be unavailable due to the disaster.

Unique ethical and legal issues can arise. In telephone consultation, for example, when the clinician cannot see the patient face-to-face, is it appropriate to make diagnoses and recommendations without visual observation of the patient, which is part of a thorough psychiatric examination? Questions can arise regarding the completeness of the telepsychiatric clinician's deciding about treatment recommendations without evaluating the patient in person. Ensuring patient confidentiality may be difficult because of lack of security on some telecommunications, increased access of federal intelligence agencies to telecommunications, and possible "hackers." Licensure and regulatory status of potential telepsychiatric clinicians presents problems because:

1. The clinician is not seeing or able to physically examine the patient.
2. State laws vary.
3. Malpractice carriers tend not to cover telepsychiatry.
4. Some states require licensure to use telepsychiatry with patients in that state.

It is important for clinicians and health agencies to contact their state licensing board and regulatory agencies before initiating telepsychiatric services.[16] This is preferably done as part of pre-disaster planning but also in the acute response if it is feasible (e.g., professional licensing board can still be contacted).

Access to the use of telepsychiatry may be influenced by cultural, language, ethnic, and socioeconomic issues, as well as physical disabilities. Some cultures may not be as receptive to the use of telepsychiatry; that is, not seeing a "real" person in a face-to-face interaction. There may be a need for translators. There may also be challenges to the use of telepsychiatry in working with individuals who have disabilities, such as visual and hearing impairments.

Administratively, organizational buy-in to telepsychiatry will be necessary. This can be especially problematic as the mechanism(s) of reimbursement for telepsychiatry is not clear for many states or in federal health programs. Acceptance of this new mode of collaborating in and providing care can also be accomplished with more research regarding the effectiveness of disaster telepsychiatry, thereby growing its evidence base.

Next Steps

There are no guidelines yet on the use of telepsychiatry in disasters. However, a paradigm of planning and using disaster telepsychiatry can be extrapolated from similar planning for general emergency telepsychiatry.[16] The implementation of disaster telepsychiatry will require multilevel approaches: individual clinician, organization, and system. For you at the level of the clinician, there will first need to be training in basic post-disaster mental health issues. Non-psychiatric clinicians should have some familiarity with recognizing and managing acute crises so that they can best utilize the consultation with the distance psychiatric clinician, and clinicians need to be trained to become competent in the use of telepsychiatry. Clinicians should learn techniques on handling safety issues surrounding the use of telepsychiatry (e.g., what to do if a patient becomes agitated and violent). Clinicians will need to learn what ethnic, language, and cultural issues may be relevant to the process.

From an organizational perspective, psychiatry should be promoted and incorporated into disaster planning. Organizational investment is necessary to develop the information technology infrastructure to enable telepsychiatry. Protocols are needed to describe indications for and how to initiate and conduct telepsychiatric consultation. Last, there is need for an investment in research to begin to identify evidence-based best practices in disaster telepsychiatry.

Conclusion

This chapter began with you succeeding in utilizing telepsychiatry to respond more effectively to the psychiatric sequelae of a mass shooting at a mall in your rural area. This example demonstrated how a disaster and public health emergency can have significant psychiatric implications for you and your community in the context of inadequate mental health resources. Health care systems can establish feasible disaster plans before such events in order to address and to mitigate the mental health sequelae of a disaster. Telepsychiatry may prove to be one such means for rapid delivery of quality disaster mental health collaboration or care even in areas with limited resources and for helping address the surge of mental health needs that are likely to challenge primary care. Clinicians, organizations, and systems may work to develop the capacities and competence necessary for collaborative care via telepsychiatry.

References

1. Hilty DM, Yellowlees PM, Cobb HC, et al. Use of secure email and telephone psychiatric consultations to accelerate rural health care delivery. *J Tel E Health*. 2006;12:490–495.

2. De Leo D, Dello Buono M, Dwyer J. Suicide among the elderly: the long-term impact of a telephone support and assessment intervention in northern Italy. *Br J Psych*. 2002;181:226–229.

3. Sorvaniemi M, Ojanen E, Santamaki O. Telepsychiatry in emergency consultations: a follow-up study of sixty patients. *Telemed J E Health*. 2005;11:439–441.

4. Sorvaniemi M, Santamaki O. Telepsychiatry in emergency consultations. *J Telemed Telecare*. 2002;8:183–184.

5. Monnier J, Knapp RG, Fruch BC. Recent advances in telepsychiatry: an updated review. *Psych Serv*. 2003;54:1604–1609.

6. Norman S. The use of telemedicine in psychiatry. *J Psych Ment Health Nurs*. 2006;13:771–777.

7. Hyler SE, Gangure DP, Batchelder ST. Can telepsychiatry replace in-person psychiatric assessments? A review and meta-analysis of comparison studies. *CNS Spectr.* 2005;10:403–413.

8. Hilty D, Luo JS, Morache C, et al. Telepsychiatry: an overview for psychiatrists *CNS Drugs.* 2002;16:527–548.

9. Shore JH, Savin D, Orton H, et al. Diagnostic reliability of telepsychiatry in American Indian veterans. *Am J Psych.* 2007;164:115–118.

10. Frueh BC, Monnier J, Yim E, et al. A randomized trial of telepsychiatry for post-traumatic stress disorder. *J Telemed Telecare.* 2007;13:142–147.

11. Cowain T. Cognitive-behavioural therapy via videoconferencing to a rural area. *Aust NZ J Psych.* 2001;35:62–64.

12. Frueh BC, Monnier J, Grubaugh Al, et al. Therapist adherence and competence with manualized cognitive-behavioral therapy for PTSD delivered via videoconferencing technology. *Behav Mod.* 2007;31:856–866.

13. Merrell RC, Cone SW, Rafiq A. telemedicine in extreme conditions: disasters, war, remote sites. *Stud Health Tech Inform.* 2008;131:99–116.

14. Garshnek V, Burkle FM. Telecommunications systems in support of disaster medicine: applications of basic information pathways. *Ann Emerg Med.* 1999;34:213–218.

15. Reissman DB, Schreiber M, Klomp RW, et al. The virtual network supporting the front lines: addressing emerging behavioral health problems following the tsunamis of 2004. *Mil Med.* 2006;171(1):40–43.

16. Shore JH, Hilty DM, Yellowlees P. Emergency management guidelines for telepsychiatry. *Gen Hosp Psych.* 2007;29:199–206.

Liability Issues

Edward Kantor, MD

Last week at your medical school reunion dance, your friend Pepper, a family practitioner in North Carolina, told you that she had volunteered for the Red Cross after Hurricane Katrina and was thinking of trying to help out again if the opportunity arose. One of the things she was worried about last time was licensing and malpractice coverage. At that time, she worked for the university and its insurance plan had agreed to extend malpractice coverage while she volunteered. The university did not, however, agree to extend workers' compensation coverage, and it was unclear to her at the time if she would have received benefits were she injured during her tour of duty in Louisiana. Now Pepper is in private practice and hasn't yet spoken to her malpractice carrier. A friend of hers had been "federalized" through a recruiting effort by Health and Human Services and was told that they were considered a federal employee for the purposes of general liability, malpractice, and workers' compensation. You remembered that the governor of Louisiana had extended license reciprocity to medical personnel working in Louisiana after the event

- Basic legal protections are afforded to medical volunteers in disaster settings by federal and state government.

- A medical volunteer is more vulnerable professionally when responding as an individual than when responding as a member of an organized group or governmental agency.

- The liability of a leader, officer, or administrator may not be covered by provisions covering a practicing medical volunteer.

- There are legal compacts and agreements that allow medical practice across jurisdictions in disaster.

- It is important to take a realistic view of the liability and malpractice risks of those participating in disaster response and to minimize these risks.

but weren't sure if that was typical or not. After chatting with her, it occurred to you that joining an organized response group made sense, if only for minimizing your liability. So you planned to look into volunteering with either your local Medical Reserve Corps, the Red Cross, or maybe even joining a DMAT team.[1]

Overview

If you are planning to volunteer or participate in a response group's activities, it makes sense to review the liability issues and regulations specific to that organization and the laws of the community you will be operating in. That will allow you to plan ahead and make your own personal preparations. Remember that malpractice coverage for health care practitioners is different from general liability for volunteers and will vary depending on the state you work in, organizational affiliation, individual roles and activities performed, and the circumstances of the event itself. Since this topic may involve technical legal language, the Glossary of Terms (see Box 23.1) later in this chapter provides some basic definitions.

There are a number of laws set up at the federal level to protect volunteer medical responders (also known as Volunteer Health Professionals, or VHPs). The Volunteer Protection Act of 1997 (VPA) states that volunteers of nonprofit or governmental entities are protected from liability for:

Harm caused by an act or omission of the volunteer on behalf of the organization or entity if: (1) the volunteer was acting within the scope of the volunteer's responsibilities; (2) if appropriate or required, the volunteer was properly licensed, certified, or authorized by the appropriate authorities for the activities or practice in the state in which the harm occurred; (3) the harm was not caused by willful or criminal misconduct, gross negligence, reckless misconduct, or a conscious, flagrant indifference to the rights or safety of the individual; and (4) the harm was not caused by the volunteer operating a motor vehicle, vessel, aircraft, or other vehicle.[2]

Most states have enacted legislation intended to provide basic legal protections to those who render aid without compensation in emergencies and during disaster events. If you inadvertently stumble into an emergency situation and assist someone in good faith, up to the limits of your ability and training, lacking gross negligence or intentional harm, most states have "Good Samaritan" statutes that will protect you from civil suit. Unfortunately, there is wide variability from state to state, so it is well worth your while to check out the related laws for the states in which you live and practice.

Good Samaritan Acts

As an example of a "Good Samaritan" statute protecting an individual providing emergency care, California law states that:

> *No person who in good faith, and not for compensation, renders emergency care at the scene of an emergency shall be liable for any civil damages resulting from any act or omission. The scene of an emergency shall not include emergency departments and other places where medical care is usually offered.*

> —*California Good Samaritan Law Health and Safety Code §1799.102*

Although helpful in emergencies, Good Samaritan laws may not apply in the aftermath of a disaster when the emergency nature of the event has stabilized and the medical care provided is no longer urgent or emergent. Over the last 5 years or so, the federal government has encouraged states to beef up their legal protections for volunteers in order to encourage participation in disaster response activities, particularly by health care providers. Most statutes providing liability protection for volunteer health providers (VHP's) require the declaration of a disaster or a state of emergency by a governmental official such as a mayor, a governor, or the president of the United States before the protective statutes apply (see Chapter 2).[3]

There is generally an expectation that a health care provider is acting in good faith, without a charge for services, in an emergency situation and/or under substandard or unusual circumstances. Since state laws vary greatly in the area of liability, in order to ensure that you understand your protections, familiarize yourself with your own state statutes before volunteering. One example of updated state law is the Commonwealth of Virginia's Volunteers Act, which has been updated recently with the advent of new volunteer initiatives supporting disaster response activities.

Virginia Code[4]

• §2.2–3601 **Definitions:** "Volunteer in state and local services shall include, but shall not be limited to, any person who serves in a **Medical Reserve Corps (MRC)** unit or on a **Community Emergency Response Team (CERT)** while engaged in emergency services and preparedness activities as defined in §44–146.16."

• §2.2–3602 **Status of Volunteers** "D. Individuals involved in emergency services and preparedness activities ... shall be considered volunteers in state and local services and shall be accordingly entitled to the benefits conferred in this chapter. ... [S]uch individuals shall be deemed to be regular-service volunteers."

• §2.2–3605 **Volunteer Benefits** "D. Liability insurance may be provided by the department utilizing their services both to regular-service and occasional-service volunteers to the same extent as may be provided by the department to its paid staff. Volunteers in state and local service, including, but not limited to, any person who serves in a **Medical Reserve Corps (MRC)** unit or on a **Community Emergency Response Team (CERT)**, shall enjoy the protection of the Commonwealth's sovereign immunity to the same extent as paid staff."

Specific Agency Coverage

For non-governmental organizations, coverage varies by individual groups. The Red Cross, for example, has comprehensive general liability insurance that covers volunteers, including physicians, nurses, and licensed or certified mental health providers while they serve as agents of the Red Cross.[5] They must be registered and work under the control and supervision of authorized Red Cross staff and following the agency's policies. At this time physicians are not authorized to prescribe medications when working under the auspices of the Red Cross.

Out-of-State Response

Volunteers and state resources that respond to disasters in another state are typically covered by an agreement dating back to 1996, the

Emergency Management Assistance Compact (EMAC), between all 50 states, Washington, D.C., and some U.S. territories. More information can be found at their web site: **www.emacweb.org**. Most of these protections do not apply to unaffiliated volunteers.

Emergency Management Assistance Compact

"**Officers or employees of a party state** rendering aid in another state pursuant to this compact **shall be considered agents of the requesting state for tort liability and immunity purposes;** and **no party state or its officers or employees** rendering aid in another state pursuant to this compact **shall be liable on account of any act or omission in good faith** on the part of such forces while so engaged **or on account of the maintenance or use of any equipment or supplies** in connection therewith. Good faith in this article shall not include willful misconduct, gross negligence, or recklessness."[6]

Federalized Volunteer Health Professionals (VHPs)

The Stafford Act gives federal agencies the power to appoint temporary personnel in the event of a public health emergency or disaster. Appointees are considered employees of the U.S. government for the purpose of liability and workers' compensation.[7] The federal and state avenues for deployment of volunteers offer different degrees of legal protections for the volunteers themselves. Table 23.1 outlines the legal protections available for volunteers deployed by the federal government under ESF-8 (the health component of disaster support activities) and EMAC.

Leadership

Individual liability is a slightly different issue than the overall risk management concerns of an organization. There can be situations where specific laws are set up to protect the individual responder who acts to help someone, but the organization she works under may not be similarly protected from liability. In addition if you serve as an officer or leader in a response group, you may not be protected in the same ways for actions or inactions you take on behalf of your organization. Ensure

Table 23.1 Legal Protections Available for Volunteer Health Personnel Under ESF-8 and EMAC

	Licensure Waivers	Liability Protections	Workers' Compensation	Reemployment Protection
Federal Intermittent Disaster Response Personnel —NDMS	Yes	Yes	Yes	Yes
Federal Temporary Employees— Schedule A, Excepted Service	Yes	Yes	Yes	No
State Volunteers Under EMAC	Yes, with VSA	Yes, with VSA	Yes with VSA	Dependent on state law

As indicated by the table above, all three avenues of deployment offer similar levels of volunteer protection. Both federal avenues provide licensure waivers, libability protections, and workers' compensation coverage. However, only federal volunteers deployed as intermittent disaster response personnel with the PHS will enjoy reemployment protection. State volunteers under EMAC may also enjoy reemployment protection, depending on the law of the state by which the volunteer is deployed. Additionally, under EMAC, the availability of all four types of legal protections will only be available if the volunteer has executed a VSA with the state by which he or she is deployed. Thus, the strength of the legal protections from states will be dependent on the terms of the VSA.

Source: Center for Law and the Public's Health. Hurricane Katrina response: incorporation of local assets into a state emergency management assistance compact (EMAC) response. Available at: **http://www.publichealthlaw.net/ Research/PDF/Katrina%20-%20Deployment%20of%20VHPs%20EMAC%20and%20ESF-8.pdf**. Accessed March 8, 2009.

that the group's liability insurance covers you as a response leader in cases of non-medical activities such as an illegal or harmful act by a volunteer reporting to you.

International Liability Issues

International disaster response activities present a host of different legal issues above those occurring within the boundaries of the United States. Some countries are extremely grateful and make the process simple. Others, with political agendas, different cultures, and varying health standards, are likely to pose more challenges to your efforts and perhaps even impact your practice options and liability. Many countries participate in pacts that protect disaster responders from liability and offer them forms of immunity similar to that given to diplomats for their responding personnel. These protections are not universal and depend upon the goodwill of the country of origin and the host nation. Volunteers from NGOs do not typically receive the same privilege.

Many organizations support organized international efforts and each has its own guidelines on liability and malpractice. Do not assume that by joining a well-known response group all of your medical activities are either covered automatically or completely. Typically, government-sponsored programs and responses under non-governmental organizations help to ensure that U.S. providers have permission to offer medical care in the disaster area.[7] Proper licensing authority and malpractice coverage are ultimately the individual practitioner's responsibility. Make sure that you are aware of the procedures for the region you plan to work in and your paperwork is in order before you begin practice in another country.

Altered Standards of Care in a Disaster Situation

Anyone who has worked in a disaster or a wilderness medical setting has experienced practice with limited technological support, a short medication list, and narrowed therapeutic options. Although physicians and nurses expect to triage resources and do their best to make good decisions with limited options, there is no accepted definition of what guidelines to follow in specific situations. This is an area of much discussion in both the legal and medical community and became a hot topic during the last 2 years as communities began to plan for pandemic influenza. It is likely that the medical definition and the legal definition will vary and that, unless specific guidelines are issued by state health and legal authorities, the ambiguity will endure.

Conclusion

Although much needs to be done to achieve consistent liability coverage for volunteer health professionals in disaster, there has been a lot of progress over the last few years, and many safe opportunities to volunteer exist.[8] Individual states continue to develop more comprehensive legal protections and some strong national efforts have evolved to support interstate compacts facilitating volunteerism and protecting the VHPs. In 2007, the National Conference of Commissioners on Uniform State Laws (NCCUSL) approved the Uniform Emergency Volunteer Health Practitioners Act (UEVHPA). This would evolve as an interstate agreement or compact that would establish a set of guidelines and an infrastructure for VHPs to work across state lines safely in disaster situations, including communication, screening and registration, scope of practice issues, and benefits and protections under the law.[9] As of January 2008, a number of states have begun legislative efforts to participate in the interstate agreement. This and other efforts are encouraging, suggesting that the trend is positive and medical volunteers are valued by the agencies and jurisdictions that request assistance.

Several months later you looked into the options in your home community. Based on your work needs and the fact that you live alone with pets, you decided you would be best suited to work with a group that supported your local area rather than travel nationally or internationally. You wanted very much to practice in a physician role and found that your local MRC seemed to be most appropriate with regard to time commitment, likely role in a response, as well as legal protections. You checked on your state law relating to disaster medical responders and found that in addition to the basic Good Samaritan laws, the state had recently enacted legislation limiting most general and medical liability against MRC volunteer practitioners who were working as part of a declared response activity.

Box 23.1 Glossary of Terms

Information about legal liability issues may be difficult to understand. Some legal terms that you may encounter as you address these issues with your MRC unit include:

- **Charitable immunity**—Immunity from liability granted to charitable or nonprofit organizations (varies by state)
- **Civil liability**—Being subject to liability for damages or restitution
- **Criminal liability**—Being subject to fine or imprisonment for having committed criminal acts
- **Federal protection**—The Volunteer Protection Act (VPA) of 1997. Because liability issues are handled primarily at the state level, there has been very little federal legislation that protects volunteers. However, in 1997, the VPA was passed, providing some limited immunity to volunteers.

  The VPA has some limitations:
  - Does not include acts of willful or wanton misconduct
  - Requires that the volunteers be properly licensed, certified, or otherwise authorized to perform the act
  - Requires that the volunteers act in the scope of their duties as a volunteer
  - Does not cover the operation of motorized vehicles
  - Covers volunteers for nonprofit organizations and government agencies, but it does not cover the organization or agency itself
  - Does not prohibit lawsuits; rather, it provides a potential defense for the volunteers if they are sued
  - Defines "volunteer" as someone who does not receive compensation (or anything of value exceeding $500 in lieu of compensation) for his services
  - Allows states to place additional conditions on immunity for volunteers
  - Does not specifically include or exclude medical or health volunteers

- **Immunity**—Exemption from liability or the defense of being exempt from liability
- **Indemnity**—A form of security against loss or an exemption from penalties
- **Negligence**—A specific tort that is the basis for many lawsuits. The four components that must be present consist of:
  1. **Duty of care**, a legal obligation (imposed on all) to act according to a standard of care when performing activities that could cause

Continued on next page

Box 23.1 Continued

> harm to others. There are special duties of care for medical and
> health professionals.
> 2. **Breach of duty**, or failure to act according to a reasonable stan-
>   dard of care when performing activities that could cause harm to
>   others.
> 3. **Causation**, or the determination of whether the breach of duty
>   caused loss or damage.
> 4. **Damages** refers to: 1) loss, damage, or injury caused by the breach
>   of duty; or 2) the compensation for loss, damage, or injury.
>
> - **Sovereign immunity**—Immunity of a state government or subunit of
>   a state government from suit (state governments, although not all,
>   may waive their sovereign immunity)
> - **Tort**—A wrongful act, omission, or violation of the duty of care
>   resulting in injury or damage to a person or property
> - **Vicarious liability**—The liability of a superior entity for the acts of its
>   subordinates (e.g., the liability of an organization for the actions of
>   its volunteers)

References

1. Albright MB, Hoke C, Wible J. MRC Technical Assistance Series. *Special Top-ics: Risk Management and Liability Basics for MRC Units.* Washington, DC: Medical Reserve Corps Program Office; 2006.

2. Volunteer Protection Act of 1997 (Public Law 105–19). Available at : **http://www.dot.gov/ost/ogc/PRO BONO/policydocs3.htm**. Accessed April 14, 2009.

3. Hodge JG, Jr., Gable LA, Cálves SH. Volunteer health professionals and emergencies: assessing and transforming the legal environment. *Biosecurity and Bioterrorism.* 2005;3:216–223.

4. Sections §2.2- 3601, 3602 and 3605, Code of Virginia, Legislative Informa-tion System. Available at: **http://leg1.state.va.us/000/lst/LS686462.HTM**. Accessed March 8, 2009.

5. International Federation of Red Cross and Red Crescent Societies. *Law and Legal Issues in International Disaster Response: A Desk Study.* Geneva: Interna-tional Federation of Red Cross and Red Crescent Societies; 1985.

6. Emergency Management Assistance Compact (Public Law 104–321). Avail-able at: **http://www.emacweb.org/?13**. Accessed April 14, 2009.

7. Robert T. Stafford Disaster Relief and Emergency Assistance Act (Public Law 93–288) as amended, June 2007. Available at: **http://www.fema.gov/about/ stafact.shtm**. Accessed March 8, 2009.

8. Peterson CA. Be safe, be prepared: emergency system for advance registration of volunteer health professionals in disaster response. *Online J Issues Nurs.* 2006.

9. Hodge JG. Legal issues concerning volunteer health professional and the hurricane-related emergencies in the Gulf Coast region. *Public Health Reports.* 2006;121:205–207.

Ethics

Joseph P. Merlino, MD, MPA

Overheated patients were dying around her, and only a few could be taken away by helicopter—the only means of escape for the most fragile patients until the water receded. Medicines were running low and, with no electricity, patients living on machines were running out of battery power. In the chaos, Dr. Pou was left to care for many patients she did not know. But did she cross a line during those harrowing days, using lethal injections to kill several patients who were in extreme distress? The attorney general of Louisiana says Dr. Pou did cross a line, and recommended that she be prosecuted for murder.[1]

Introduction

Hurricane Katrina's assault on New Orleans provided a glimpse of possibly unimaginable ethical dilemmas faced by local health care providers. While charges against Dr. Pou were later dropped, it was only after a protracted legal battle in which these care givers were alleged to have committed euthanasia. Did you ever think about what you would do in such situations?

- Ethical dilemmas and conflicts don't have easy answers or solutions.

- It is strongly recommended that individuals and health care organizations practice disaster drills to appropriately prepare themselves and their institutions for a variety of disaster scenarios; these drills should include time for ethical reflection and discussion.

- Professional organizations for various health care providers have a code of ethics that can often be found on the Internet and can be helpful in thinking about resolution of dilemmas.

This chapter looks at some of the ethical issues confronted by primary care first responders during the initial days of a disaster response. As the duration of a disaster response goes on, more systems will presumably return to their pre-disaster routine operational status and the ethical issues applicable will likewise return to pre-disaster mode.[2,3]

Confidentiality and Professional Boundaries

Two potential ethical concerns for health care providers responding to disasters are issues of confidentiality and the maintenance of appropriate professional boundaries. Let's look at actual clinical situations from the first response to the 9/11 attacks in New York City as examples of this issue.

Called to assist a firehouse team who lost members of their company during 9/11, I quickly found myself in situations where information was being given to me, and asked of me, about some of the firefighters believed to be in need of mental health attention for a variety of reasons, including:

- New members ("probees") lacking support and feeling isolated from their "brothers"
- "Super-macho" attitudes in some of the firefighters who refused to take any time off and were feared to be "burning out"
- Excessive use of alcohol to numb feelings of loss and to induce sleep

My role suddenly became that of "house-psychiatrist." Improvising as best I could to meet the clinical demands, I set up my office in one of the firehouse bedrooms and held group sessions in the firehouse kitchen. There was no record-keeping. Professional neutrality was challenged by the physical setting described above and by the fact that, while I was the professional caregiver, I too was impacted by the terrorist attacks and this was hard to conceal as the long hours and stress took their toll on me as well as the firefighters I was there to help.

Intuitively, the working model that I found myself using is what I now call "the medical neighbor model."[4] This approach is comparable to that of the physician who has a very close family member, or good friend and neighbor, who is seriously ill. The medical-neighbor model is applicable to many first responders, regardless of specialty. The doctor in this scenario is not "*the*" doctor but an informed and caring participant, who is *a doctor*, simultaneously impacted by the neighbor or relative's medical crisis. Adopting this approach enabled me the freedom to have the feelings I had without guilt, to walk away when I needed to, to share my sadness openly, and to be as much a neighbor or brother or son as a doctor. Confidentiality was maintained with disclosures permitted in cases of dangerousness to self or others, as in non-disaster situations.

In this role I could still draw upon my medical and psychiatric skills to identify individuals in need of traditional medical care and referral. Utilizing my "medical neighbor" role allowed me to make such a referral while simultaneously advocating for and facilitating this referral. This model allows for any unavoidable boundary crossings during a first response to a disaster (e.g., using a bedroom to do clinical exam or lending or giving money). This should not to be confused with inappropriate boundary violations (e.g., sexual). Recall that a boundary violation is a boundary crossing that is exploitative—it gratifies the doctor's need at the expense of the patient.[5]

Providing Comfort and Avoiding Sexual Boundary Violations

Let's look now at another area of ethical concern you may be confronted with during your disaster response, that pertaining to boundary violations. Boundary violations, including intimate touching and frank sexual contact, are more likely to occur in individuals who are themselves stressed and emotionally deprived.[6,7] The natural urge to comfort someone in distress can include a seemingly harmless hug, which can be experienced as inappropriate physical and sexual contact. To protect against possible boundary violations in disaster settings it is important to pay careful attention to fulfilling *your own* emotional needs in ways that do not jeopardize the professional relationship with those you are caring for. Interacting in generally open and more public spaces instead of in closed or out of the way offices adds another level of protection to ensure a respect for professional boundary keeping. Further information on the topic of self-care is available in Chapter 3.

Your Role Does *Not* Include "Fitness for Duty" Evaluations

Another issue that came up during 9/11, and will come up in future disaster responses, is the issue of assessing "fitness for duty" while assisting members of the uniformed services, including police and fire personnel. This can be challenging and may be difficult at times for the clinician who is pressed by others to make such a determination. It should be noted that fitness evaluations are typically made by agents of the employer (e.g., the police department or the fire department) and not the individual's primary mental health provider, or in the case of a disaster, by you. In the 9/11 vignette above, the fire department did indeed have its own representatives who made these decisions for their personnel. By asking the officer in charge, the correct contact can be identified and notified.

Record Keeping

The matter of record keeping is another potential ethical dilemma for the first responder. While typical record keeping would not occur, a confidential log should be kept including the minimal necessary information. This information should include, at a minimum, the individual's name, location, date seen, risk assessment, any medications prescribed, and contact information for follow-up if needed. Similarly, those individuals cared for should receive your contact information in the event they wish to make contact later, including after the disaster. This happened after the 9/11 attacks in New York City when individuals receiving emotional first aid declined further treatment initially but sought it several months after 9/11.

Ethical Aspects in Assessing Dangerousness

As in non-disaster settings, an assessment finding dangerousness to self or others should prompt transport to a hospital emergency room for further evaluation and admission as indicated. But in a disaster, when is "dangerousness to self" ethically acceptable, if ever? What if someone was exposed to a chemical or biological agent known to have a high mortality rate? Should this individual be allowed to commit suicide as a rational act of autonomy? Clearly, such a situation might be one of your worst nightmares. How would, or should, you respond to such a request? Determinations about one's right to "rational suicide" must include a thorough evaluation of the individual's mental status. Specifically, is this person suffering from any mental or medical illness that is compromising his capacity to assess his clinical condition, recommended treatment, and prognosis? Does he fully understand this information and is he able to process it in a manner consistent with his long-held values? Clearly the safest course is temporization—providing a safe setting in which the individual can take the time to reflect on his decision and contact, if possible, family or loved ones to participate in the discussion and possibly the decision.

Ethical Issues in Triage

Another ethical challenge occurs when resources are dramatically limited. In such scenarios, how should triage be conducted? Who should be cared for and who should be left untreated, possibly left to die? The opening case of this chapter gives us a glimpse of just such a situation, becoming a flashpoint during Hurricane Katrina in New Orleans when some frail elderly persons died in a hospital that was being evacuated and a physician and two nurses were arrested and charged with homicide.[8] James F. Childress discusses triage issues addressing criteria for rationing scarce resources. He notes what *should not* be considered in triage decisions. Factors that *should not* be considered in allocating resources include age, ethnicity, gender, disabilities or deformities, socioeconomic status, substance abuse, or aggressive behaviors. Rather, according to Childress, morally justifiable triage criteria include the likelihood of benefit, the effect on improving the quality of life, the duration of the benefit, and the urgency of the need.[9] These are clearly tough decisions to have to make, but Childress's guidelines offer some ethically sound assistance to making them.

Performance-Enhancing Medications

As our culture and the subculture of health care change, so do the ethical dilemmas with which we as health care providers are confronted. The issue of "brain enhancement" medications is one such example.[10]

Given the need for sustained and focused attention as well as endurance and stamina, should disaster responders take advantage of the medicinal effects of pharmacological agents like Adderall (amphetamine and dextroamphetamine), a stimulant, and Provigil (modafinil), which promotes wakefulness? Military researchers have focused their attention on the drug modafinil, as an alternative to amphetamines, to limit mental fatigue among military personnel so that human error such as death by "friendly fire" can be reduced.[11]

One user who posted an anonymous message about the use of brain-enhancing medications on the Chronicle of Higher Education web site, wrote:

> *I'm not talking about being able to work longer hours without sleep (although that helps), I'm talking about being able to take on twice the responsibility, work twice as fast, write more effectively, manage better, be more attentive, devise better and more creative strategies.*[10]

With this kind of endorsement, should such medications be part of our routine disaster preparedness? Who would argue that being more effective, attentive, and creative while needing less sleep during a disaster response isn't a desirable goal? But is it ethical? Author Francis Fukuyama notes in his book *Our Posthuman Future: Consequences of the Biotechnology Revolution*: "The original purpose of medicine is to heal the sick, not turn healthy people into gods."

Fukuyama's statement begs the question: Should the same rules, norms, ethics that apply during "normal" times also apply during times of crises and disaster? Or is this a slippery slope that ought not to be traveled? The dilemma which Dr. Pou faced at the beginning of this chapter suggests the kind of terrible ethical dilemma a clinician might face in a disaster, and quite separately, so does the temptation of clinicians using medications to enhance attention, concentration, and endurance at such times.

Conclusion

Ethical dilemmas and conflicts may not have easy answers or solutions. Confronting them in the midst of a disaster for the first time is a situation most of us would hope to avoid. Situations are rarely "black or white." By increasingly adding confounders to your disaster drill ("what if" scenarios), you and your organization can be helpfully stretched to think and plan for the unthinkable. Such preparation will make it more likely that if confronted with an ethical challenge during an actual disaster, you may be better prepared having thought about how to navigate a path not previously taken and being aware of where to turn for helpful resources on ethical principles and practice.

Professional organizations for various health care providers have codes of ethics that can help you as you prepare. (See Box 24.1.) Such codes reflect the consensus about the general standards of appropriate professional conduct and are often found on the Internet.[5] You are advised to review your discipline's code of ethics now as you are thinking about this aspect of preparedness (and while you have electricity and access to the Internet). These principles offer guidance to approaching potential ethical dilemmas you may face during disaster response.

Remember our colleague Peter who we introduced to you earlier in this volume? Peter reacted with panic to a disaster mobilization call—not sure whether to report or to stay home with his son and pregnant wife. What if Peter chose to stay at home and not report? Would he have acted ethically?

Much has been written about first responders, physicians, and other health professionals' obligations to participate in disasters and catastrophes. But what is owed to health professionals as they prepare and also engage in longer-term actions geared to protect their community's and nation's health and well-being?[3] I would argue that physicians are duty-bound by their professional values to medically assist in times of disaster. But what form and manner this assistance takes must be shaped by the individual physician's life and personal values.

Box 24.1 Codes of Ethics

- The American Medical Association's Code of Ethics:
  http://www.ama-assn.org/ama/pub/category/2498.html
- The American Nurses Association Code of Ethics:
  http://nursingworld.org/mods/mod580/cecde03.htm
- The National Association of Social Workers:
  http://www.utexas.edu/ssw/aa/forms/resources/codes.pdf

As has been stated many times already in this text, preparation *before-hand* is the key to optimal action. Before, not during, is the best time for the community of citizens to weigh-in, for example, on whether or not individual liberties should yield to the needs of the community or nation, and if so, how and to what extent. Should the states enact an Emergency Health Powers Act similar to the one initially developed by the Center for Law and the Public's Health at Georgetown and Johns Hopkins Universities? This model law empowered public health authorities with broad powers, including mandatory testing, treatment and vaccinations programs, isolation and quarantine powers, and imposition of travel restrictions.[12] This law is based on the precedent that protecting the public's health during an emergency, even at the risk of infringing upon the individual's civil liberties, is an essential goal of government. Debating what, if any, checks and balances should exist had best occur before, not during, an actual disaster.

References

1. Drew C, Dewan S. Louisiana doctor said to have faced chaos. *New York Times.* July 20, 2006.

2. For an excellent review of many of the ethical issues involved in disaster and post-disaster response, which are beyond the scope of this text, see *In the Wake of Terror: Medicine and Morality in a Time of Crisis* edited by Jonathan D. Moreno (see references 9 and 12).

3. Eckenwiler LA. Ethical issues in emergency preparedness and response for health professionals. *Virtual Mentor: AMA J Ethics.* 2004;6:5:1–6.

4. Merlino JP. The other Ground Zero. In: Katz CL, Pandya A, Eds. *Disaster Psychiatry: When Nightmares Come True.* New York, NY: The Analytic Press; 2004:31–36.

5. Sadock BJ, Sadock VA. *Kaplan and Sadock's Synopsis of Psychiatry.* 10th ed. Philadelphia, PA: Lippincott Williams & Wilkins; 2007.

6. Council on Ethical and Judicial Affairs. Report A– I-90: Sexual Misconduct in the Practice of Medicine. Available at: **http://www.ama-assn.org/ama1/pub/upload/mm/369/ceja_ai90.pdf**. Accessed 3/9/09.

7. Kardener SH. Sex and the physician-patient relationship. *Am J Psychiatr.* 1974;131:1134–1136.

8. Curiel TJ. Perspective: Murder or mercy? Hurricane Katrina and the need for disaster training. *N Engl J Med.* 2006;355:2067–2069.

9. Childress JF. Triage in response to a bioterrorist attack. In: Moreno JD, Ed. *In the Wake of Terror: Medicine and Morality in a Time of Crisis.* Cambridge, MA: MIT Press; 2003:77–94.

10. Carey B. Brain enhancement is wrong, right? *New York Times.* March 9, 2008:1.

11. Moreno JD. Juicing the brain. *Scientific American.* November 29, 2006.

12. Moreno JD, Ed. *In the Wake of Terror: Medicine and Morality in a Time of Crisis.* Cambridge, MA: MIT Press; 2003.

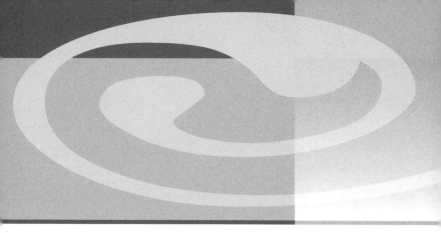

PART

5

Epilogue

Section Editor: Joseph P. Merlino, MD, MPA

Life After the Disaster: Follow-Up, Resilience, and Recovery

Knight Aldrich, MD, Joseph P. Merlino, MD, MPA, Craig L. Katz, MD, and Frederick J. Stoddard, Jr., MD

Personal Reflections

Peter thought that he would nap on the way home, but although he was tired—as he had been for practically the entire time he had been at the site—he found that he just couldn't sleep. He was glad—overjoyed, he told himself—that he was on his way home, and there was no doubt about his looking forward to seeing his family, friends, patients, and practice associates. He had missed them all, and one of the frustrations about his recent disaster work was the difficulty in communication; mail was uncertain, email often didn't function, telephones were out a lot of the time, and his cell phone behaved erratically. He also ran out of batteries. He had not brought many with him because he thought there would be plenty there. With the utilities knocked out, batteries were at a premium. That's one thing he would recommend to the next volunteer: Bring more batteries than you think you'll ever need!

Another recommendation for future volunteers concerned money. In the disaster area no one had enough money. The banks were not open and no one would cash his checks. It wasn't that they did not trust him but because there wasn't any way to cash them. He'd actually brought along a lot of cash, but he realized that

- Take the time to reflect on what you have just experienced and about what lies ahead as you return to your *normal* life.

- Consider if your disaster work has changed your view of medical practice and mental health care.

- While medicine often focuses on disease and illness, what have you learned about human characteristics like fortitude, versatility, and altruism?

- Would you do this again?

may have been a mistake—it made him the only one with the ability to pick up the check! He found himself sometimes resenting this role when he thought that his paying for things was being taken for granted by some. He thought that maybe he should have taken less cash, but then he would feel a bit ashamed because so many of the people he helped out financially had lost everything they had.

His health was fine—better than at home, really—because he ate less, got more exercise from all of the running around, and he actually lost a few pounds. Generally he was pleased that he had adapted so well to primitive facilities; it reminded him of going to summer camp as a kid. Another thing besides cash and batteries that he'd advise others to bring was laundry soap and nutrition bars.

Practicing Medicine

In some ways Peter imagined that the disaster duty was like a locum tenens assignment in a primitive culture. In other ways, though, it was totally different. He had made much more of a commitment here than he thought he ever would make to a locum tenens job. In fact, at one point he found himself overcommitted; for several days in a row when he was almost alone he had gotten up early and worked late, missed meals, and never got off his feet. He had been warned about the need to take care of himself, but he was so concerned about all the people he felt responsible for that he just kept going until he was totally exhausted. Finally another doctor showed up, took one look at him, and told him he had to take some time off. He would not be able to continue doing what he came for if he didn't. He had such a feeling of commitment before, but with individual patients; he'd never felt so committed to a whole community that needed him. It was perhaps the only time in his life he felt so needed. While it was rewarding, almost exhilarating, he knew that it couldn't last. Peter did not expect this. He was lucky that the other doctor showed up when he did or he might have had to come home early, which would have been terribly disappointing to him.

There was another big difference from an ordinary locum assignment where the patients and everybody else were going about their business in the usual way. It was the attachments he had developed, not only to the people he treated and the ones who helped him, but to just about everybody. Before he arrived Peter thought that he would be counting the days until he could get back home, but as the time of departure came closer he felt real sadness and grief as he anticipated leaving so many people he had grown to love and admire. He knew intellectually that he would soon get over these feelings and probably would never write or phone any of the people he met, but at this time they were very important to him.

That probably contributed to his frustration at not knowing how the treatment he was providing would turn out. He wasn't used to having so little back-up—X-rays, sophisticated lab studies, scans, all the paraphernalia he had become convinced was essential to practice good medicine. It was a real satisfaction to find that he could practice good medicine in spite of not having the latest technologies. He was glad that he had gotten a little head start by taking a rural medicine elective in family medicine during medical school.

That doesn't mean that everything went well. He found that caring for patients with insulin-dependent diabetes with no lab and without insulin supplies was scary, but he muddled through. The patients certainly appreciated his efforts. It also was very tough, espcially when he had to improvise when no drug stores were open or when there was no refrigeration. He thought of adding a *Physician's Desk Reference* (PDR) to the list of stuff he should have brought with him but decided that it was not only too heavy but also frustrating to look up drug after drug that wasn't available.

Peter knew he would be happy to see his regular patients again and to be back in his usual professional routine. But he had a sense that the usual pace of things would lack the excitement of what he had just done, and he wondered whether he would be bored. Peter had become a physician because he thrived on helping people, but there was really not too much heroism involved in the daily grind of practice he had been accustomed to before his disaster work.

Psychiatric Complaints

There were more patients with psychiatric complaints than he had anticipated, and without drugs he couldn't do much but listen to them. He was amazed at what just listening seemed to accomplish and even found that most of the time when he stopped listening and gave advice things didn't go nearly as well. He could not listen indefinitely, however. Peter had to limit his sessions in time and relied on his watch to limit "talking visits" (and that reminded him that a spare watch battery should be included in the volunteer's baggage, or better yet, bring the old fashioned wind-up kind).

Peter hadn't heard of psychological first aid before, and when he first did he thought it was a restatement of the obvious. Medical first aid—that was something substantive. However, he quickly realized that the simplicity of the principles of psychological first aid were what made them so useful—he could actually learn and apply them while engaged in providing medical care. One clinic even had put a typed copy of them up on the wall.

He was surprised at the resilience of the "psych" patients and their high apparent recovery rate. It made him less pessimistic than he had been in his practice about such patients. He also learned from the psychiatrist that occasionally consulted with him how to cope with—really how to treat—hypochondriacs and he was eager to put what he had learned into practice at home. Instead of ordering a bunch of tests and trying to persuade these patients that the tests showed that their symptoms were psychological, he now would tell them (after he had interviewed them but before any tests were done) that he felt sure that the causes of the symptoms were psychological but that he would order some tests to make sure that there was nothing organic in addition to the psychological going on. And then he would listen for a short time to the patients' concerns about their life situations and schedule a few weekly short visits.

He had learned, too, to spot depression better and also to consider more often clinical depression and post-traumatic stress disorder besides cardiac or other kinds of organic illnesses when the symptoms justified it. All in all, Peter had learned a lot about himself as well as about practicing medicine.

Ready for Another?

Would he volunteer again? When Peter first arrived and was overwhelmed by it, all he thought was "never again," but as time passed and he began to feel better about his ability to cope, his view changed. He thought about volunteering, not next week or next month, but next year? Probably, he thought. If he could get his friends to cover for him again, although they weren't all that enthusiastic about covering this time. They did it, but they seemed to think he was a little odd to want to volunteer. He wondered how much to tell them about his disaster experience. He thought about offering to give a talk at the county medical society and grand rounds at his hospital.

Did he say a year from now he would be ready? Peter had forgotten that, if all went as planned, he and his wife would have a baby by then. Maybe he ought to wait until the baby is 3 years old and at least past the "terrible twos." In fact, Peter realized that he better think about making it up to Susie for being away so long before he even thought about more disaster duty. Or, he laughed, he would have his own private disaster right at home!

Conclusion

This book has aimed to share basic knowledge of mental health for primary care clinicians in disasters. After the Introduction, there are four parts, followed by this Epilogue and a supplement on Resources. Peter is the primary care clinician protagonist in many chapters, which are filled with actual examples with a practical or "real world" quality.

Part 1, Preparation, addresses how one becomes involved in disaster response, ways of communicating (Chapter 5, Risk Communication, Prevention, and the Media) with the public and the media about health risk and safety, practical steps to take while preparing to volunteer to work in a disaster (Chapter 4, Roughing It), Caring for one's own and one's family's emotions (Chapter 3, Self-Care), and making sense of and utilizing the many agencies and elements in the Disaster Response System in the United States.(Chapter 2, The Disaster Response System in the United States).

Part 2, Assessment, begins with consideration for how to differentiate normal responses to the stress of a disaster from those which may reflect psychopathology and how to obtain psychiatric consultation when necessary. This leads naturally into a discussion of identification of those at risk (Chapter 7, Assessment and Management of Suicidality After Disasters), including use of screening tools (Chapter 8, Screening for Mental Health Issues Following Disaster) to identify those with symptoms of greatest concern who may require more and potentially rapid intervention. Next, the plight of developing children in the disaster setting is discussed, again supporting use of brief questionnaires to identify problems, as well as providing parental and family supports to lessen the child's distress (Chapter 9, Children and Families). Another key area of potential problems is those with medically unexplained symptoms (MUPS) who may overwhelm emergency services and who must be triaged, clinically evaluated as appropriate, and followed-up with over time (Chapter 10, Medically Unexplained Symptoms). Other subpopulations meriting focused assessment are women, minorities, those with severe and persistent mental illness, the elderly, the economically disadvantaged, and the homeless (Chapter 11, Difficult Encounters and Chapter 12, Special Populations in Disaster). And many presenting for medical care following disasters are experiencing bereavement (Chapter 13, Bereavement and Disasters). The example of Shakespeare's Macduff illustrates the disbelief, grief, and hopelessness typical after the loss of one's children and family as well as the potential benefit of being unburdened of such feelings of grief.

Part 3, Intervention, deals with ways to address problems. Psychological first aid, in some ways like the "stopping the bleeding" of physical first aid, seeks to mitigate the impact of traumatic events by providing acute psychological support, emotional nurturance, and hope to those most impacted (Chapter 14, Psychological First Aid). Working with responders is key, as they are among those most at risk for suffering the adverse consequences of trauma (Chapter 15, Understanding and Helping Responders). Social interventions strengthen or provide family, community, educational, religious, or economic resources and are critical to resilience in the face of disaster (Chapter 16, Social Interventions in Disaster). Psychological interventions provide reassurance and hope, reduce stress, support coping, facilitate grieving, provide stepped services geared to the problems, and improve outcomes (Chapter 17, Psychological Interventions). When judiciously used, despite a limited evidence base, psychopharmacological interventions may also facilitate recovery, especially from acute manifestations of acute stress, anxiety, or depression (Chapter 18, Psychopharmacology). Collaborative care with mental health professionals can be an essential resource to assist the mental health assessment and interventions conducted by primary care clinicians, from triage to more focused interventions and dispositions, including hospitalization for mental disorders or substance abuse (Chapter 19, Collaborative Care). Staff support addresses the entire disaster community and requires anticipatory preparation and ongoing triage, diagnosis, brief interventions, and formal treatment when appropriate (Chapter 20, Staff Support). International perspectives reflect how work abroad entails very different relief agencies, cultural and socioeconomic conditions, pre-disaster population risks, resources, and goals (Chapter 21, International Disaster Perspectives).

In Special Issues, Part 4, special issues are presented in the context of disaster response, and a few issues important to the primary care clinician are presented as well. Telebehavioral health is an exciting emerging area, allowing more collaboration with mental health professionals at a distance (Chapter 22, Telepsychiatry). Every health professional working in disaster response should be aware of the liability issues pertinent to this unique work (Chapter 23, Liability Issues). Similarly, the ethics of disaster situations should be anticipated in preparing for and providing health services to various disaster-impacted populations (Chapter 24, Ethics).

Resources

Chapter 1: Getting Involved

Uniformed Service Agencies and Organizations

National Guard: http://www.1800goguard.com/careers/index.php
Public Health Service Commissioned Corps: http://www.usphs.gov/

Civilian Organizations

American Red Cross (ARC): http://www.redcross.org
Civilian Medical Reserve Corps (MRC): http://www.medical
reservecorps.gov
Computer Emergency Readiness Team (CERT): http://www.citizen
corps.gov/cert/
National Disaster Medical System (NDMS): http://www.hhs.gov/
aspr/opeo/ndms/index.html
Remote Area Medical (RAM): http://www.ramusa.org/

Disaster Volunteer Agencies and Clearinghouses

AMA Center for Disaster Preparedness: http://www.ama-assn.org/
ama/pub/physician-resources/public-health/center-public-health-
preparedness-disaster-response.shtml
Alliance for Information and Referral Systems (AIRS): http://www
.airs.org
America's Fraternal Benefit Organizations: http://www.nfcanet.org
Association For Volunteer Administration (AVA): http://www
.avaintl.org
Citizen Corps: http://www.citizencorps.gov
City Cares of America: http://www.citycares.org

Corporation for National and Community Service: http://www
.nationalservice.org

Disaster Volunteers: http://www.disastervolunteers.org/

Emergency Management Assistance Compact (EMAC): http://www
.emacweb.org/

Federal Emergency Management Agency (FEMA): http://www.fema.gov

Help In Disaster: http://www.helpindisaster.org

Humane Society of the United States: http://www.hsus.org

International Association of Emergency Managers (IAEM):
http://www.iaem.com

International Association of Fire Chiefs (IAFC): http://www.iafc.org

National Association of Planning Councils: http://www.community
planning.org

National Emergency Management Association (NEMA): http://www
.nemaweb.org

National Voluntary Organizations Active In Disaster (NVOAD):
http://www.nvoad.org

Points of Light Foundation and Volunteer Center National Network:
http://www.pointsoflight.org

The Salvation Army: http://www.usn.salvationarmyusa.org

United Way of America: http://www.unitedway.org

The UPS Foundation: http://www.community.ups.com

U.S. Chamber of Commerce: http://www.uschamber.com

USA Freedom Corps: http://www.usafreedomcorps.gov

USA Initiative: http://www.usa.pointsoflight.org

Volunteer Center National Network: http://www.1800volunteer.org

World Cares: http://worldcares.org

Chapter 10: Medically Unexplained Physical Symptoms

Screening Tools

Idiopathic Physical Symptoms: PHQ-15

Kronke K, Spitzer RL, Williams JB. The PHQ-15: validity of a new
measure for evaluating the severity of somatic symptoms. *Psychosom
Med.* 2002;64(2);258–266.

Psychiatric Distress: BSI-18

Derogatis LR. *Brief Symptom Inventory-18: Administration, Scoring, and Procedures Manual.* Minneapolis: Pearson; 2000.

Psychiatric Disorders: PRIME-MD

Spitzer RL, Kroenke K, Williams. Validation and utility of a self-report version of PRIME-MD: the PHQ primary care study. *JAMA.* 1999; 282:18:1737–1744.

PTSD Symptom Scale: Interview Version

Foa EB, Tolin DF. Comparison of the PTSD symptom scale: interview version and the clinician-administered PTSD scale. *J Traumatic Stress.* 2000;13(2):181–191.

PTSD Checklist Scale

Ventureyra VA, Yao SN, Cottraux J, Note I, De Mey-Guillanrd C. The validation of the post-traumatic stress disorder checklist scale in post-traumatic stress disorder and nonclinical subjects. *Psychother Psychosom.* 2002;71(1):47–53.

Worry About Illness and Conviction: Whitely Index, Illness Attitudes Scale, Somatosensory Amplification Scale

Speckens AE, Van Hemert AM, Spinhoven P, Bolk JH. The diagnostic and prognostic significance of the Whitely Index, the Illness Attitude Scales and the Somatosensory Amplification Scale. *Psychol Med.* 1996;26(5):1085–90.

Other tools may also be useful. See Figure 1, "Candidate Assessment Tools for Possible Triage Process Use" located in: Engel CC, Locke S, Reissman DB, DeMartino R, Kutz I, McDonald M, Barsky AJ. Terrorism, trauma and mass casualty triage: how might we solve the latest mind-body problem? *Biosecurity and Bioterrorism: Biodefense Strategy, Practice, and Science.* 2007; 5(2):1–9.

Chapter 18: Psychopharmacology

Drug Effects and Drug Reactions Internet Sources

A great free website to visit is **http://www.rxlist.com**. Type the name of the drug in the search box on the main page, select the drug from the list of results, and click on side effects and drug interactions on the left-hand column for that drug. Use the professional tab since there is also a consumer tab.

Another database, subscription only, is **http://www.lexi.com**; it is very easy to navigate. Click on Lexi-Comp ONLINE Login on top right corner of page and enter user name and password.

Book Sources

Lexi-Comp's *Drug Reference Handbook*. Different handbooks are available from Lexi-Comp's, such as pediatrics, adult, psychiatry, etc.

American Society of Health-System Pharmacists, *AHFS Drug Information*, 2008, 4,000 pages.

Chapter 23: Liability Issues

Resources for More Information About Liability

For more information on your state's liability laws regarding volunteers, see the Public Entity Risk Institute Publication, *State Liability Laws for Charitable Organizations and Volunteers*, 4th ed, available for download at: **http://nonprofitrisk.org/downloads/state-liability.pdf**

Centers for Disease Control and Prevention's public health law materials: **http://www2a.cdc.gov/phlp/lawmat.asp**

Health Resources and Services Administration's emergency systems for advance registration of volunteer health professionals: legal and regulatory issues: **http://www.publichealthlaw.net/Research/Affprojects .htm#HRSA**

MRC deployment information from the 2005 hurricane season: **http://www.medicalreservecorps.gov/Hurricane/DeploymentInfo**

Nonprofit Law's Volunteer Liability and the Volunteer Protection Act of 1997: **http://www.nonprofitlaw.com/quicktipsvol.shtml**

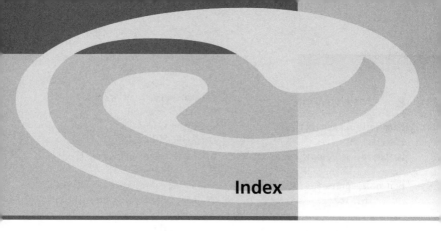

Index

Medical Society of the State of New York

Important Directions for Taking the Post Test Exam, Evaluation and to Receive Continuing Medical Education Credits for *Hidden Impact: What You Need to Know for the Next Disaster: A Practical Mental Health Guide for Clinicians*

Completion of a post-test and evaluation form are important components of this CME activity. A passing grade on the post-test is required to receive the continuing medical education credits. Please take the following test and mark your answers on the test form. Provide us your feedback by completing the evaluation form.

Physicians will need to provide their name and contact information in order for the continuing medical education credits to be awarded.

Submit the marked post-test and the completed evaluation form either by mail, fax or email to:

Medical Society of the State of New York
Public Health and Education
Attn: Sharon Damiano
1 Commerce Plaza, Suite 408
Albany, NY 12210

Fax: 1–518–465–0976

Email:
sdamiano@mssny.org

The Medical Society of the State of New York will send your certificate of participation in the course and will award you 8.0 Continuing Medical Education Credits.

The post-test exam may also be completed on-line through the Medical Society's on-line program. Physicians must register on-line at www.bcnny.com and go to the training page to the post-test exam entitled "Hidden Impact: What You Need to Know for the Next Disaster: A Practical Mental Health Guide for Clinicians." Upon successful completion of the post-test, physicians will be asked to complete an evaluation on-line. Physicians will be able to download the certificate upon completion of these steps.

The Medical Society of the State of New York is accredited by the Accreditation Council for Continuing Medical Education (ACCME) to provide continuing medical education for physicians. The Medical Society of the State of New York designates this continuing medical education activity for a maximum of 8.0 AMA PRA Category 1 Credits™. Physician should claim credit commensurate with the extent of their participation in the activity. Accredited May 2009–May 2012

Hidden Impact:
What You Need to Know for the Next Disaster:
A Practical Mental Health Guide for Clinicians
Medical Society of the State of New York

The Medical Society of the State of New York is accredited by the Accreditation Council for Continuing Medical Education (ACCME) to provide continuing medical education for physicians. The Medical Society of the State of New York designates this continuing medical education activity for a maximum of 8.0 AMA PRA Category 1 Credits™. Physician should claim credit commensurate with the extent of their participation in the activity. Accredited May 2009–May 2012

Physician Name _____

Mailing Address _____

Email address _____

(Please mail post-test to Medical Society of the State of New York, 1 Commerce Plaza, Suite 408, Albany NY 12210 or fax to Sharon Damiano at 518–465–0976)

1. All of the following are possible psychological responses to a disaster that occur within days of the event except:
   a. Insomnia
   b. Depressed mood
   c. Post-traumatic stress disorder
   d. Increased smoking
   e. Withdrawing from others

2. According to the Institute of Medicine, psychological responses to disasters and terrorism:
   a. Often involve psychiatric disorders
   b. Include changes in how people feel but not how they behave
   c. Should be the focus of our clinical attention when they are severe
   d. Involve distress, behaviors, and psychiatric disorders
   e. Are best addressed by family, friends, and clergy

3. Which is not a recommended way to address medically unexplained symptoms?
   a. Have one designated clinician assigned to the patient
   b. Focus on function rather than symptoms

    c. Explore psychosocial issues

    d. Utilize extra testing and procedures to reassure the patient

    e. Offer close follow-up

4. Which is true regarding the psychological impact of disasters on women?

    a. They are at less risk for mental health problems

    b. Women should be excused from usual domestic responsibilities

    c. Having children reduces women's trauma by distracting them

    d. They face the unique stress of being targets of violence in conflict situations

    e. They do better than men because they are more likely to seek out help

5. Suicidality is of concern in the disaster setting because:

    a. Evidence shows that suicide rates increase

    b. Survivors often question the meaning and value of life

    c. Usual risk factors for suicide do not apply amid the chaos of disaster

    d. You will be less able than usual to alter the likelihood of suicide attempts

    e. None of the above

6. When planning mental health interventions after a disaster, types of interventions to consider include:

    a. Psychological

    b. Psychopharmacological

    c. Collaborative care with mental heath professionals

    d. International

    e. All of the above

7. Psychological first aid utilizes:

    a. Debriefing

    b. Cognitive behavior therapy

    c. Modular pragmatic interventions (e.g., physical, psychological, cognitive, and spiritual)

    d. c only

    e. a, b, and c

8. Psychopharmacological interventions in acute disaster settings include which of the following:
   a. Credentialing by a medical disaster response organization such as the state department of mental health, a certified hospital or clinic, the Public Health Service, the military, or a DMAT team
   b. Obtaining a history of prior and current medications
   c. Emphasis on short-term psychotropic medications (e.g., anti-anxiety)
   d. Focus on symptoms rather than disorders
   e. All of the above

9. Early psychological interventions following trauma and disasters include:
   a. Cognitive behavioral interventions
   b. Play therapy with children and parent guidance
   c. Interventions to prevent or reduce substance abuse
   d. Psychoanalytic psychotherapy
   e. a, b, and c only

10. Which of the following statements about international perspectives on interventions is true?
    a. Health professionals are always needed and welcome at international disaster sites
    b. Ethnic and expatriate communities are at reduced risk of experiencing stigma, victimization, and mental health distress from disasters overseas
    c. Survivors of disasters have many ordinary but few unique mental health needs in the international setting
    d. All large disasters have global impacts on mental health
    e. d only

11. When volunteering your services during a disaster, which of the following is true:
    a. It is important to do whatever is asked of you, regardless of your comfort zone
    b. You should work within your general area(s) of competence
    c. Committing to multiple response groups is preferable to committing to one group
    d. All of the above
    e. a and c

12. Which of the following is true of the National Incident Management System (NIMS):
    a. NIMS is the federal infrastructure to coordinate interagency and inter-jurisdictional cooperation during a disaster event
    b. NIMS is designed to be flexible and responsive regardless of the type of disaster
    c. Under NIMS, the scale of an event determines whether it stays local or whether assistance is requested from other regional or national resources
    d. All of the above
    e. None of the above

13. Some of the selfless benefits of volunteering include which of the following:
    a. People who are generous with their time tend to live longer, happier lives
    b. The opportunity for referrals to your practice is increased
    c. Volunteering provides opportunities for celebration, courage, and humor
    d. All of the above
    e. a and c

14. Concerning the acquisition of diarrhea when traveling to a distant land for a disaster response:
    a. Risk is a minimal concern
    b. It is not usually caused by eating unwashed vegetables or fruit
    c. It can be minimized by using bottled or purified water
    d. A decontaminant like iodine is not advisable if unsure of the water source
    e. Ice need not be a concern because the water is frozen

15. Which of the following statements about risk communication are true:
    a. Risk communication refers to the use of effective communication during a crisis
    b. Fear and confusion are decreased by clear and consistent information
    c. Accurate positive communication increases one's sense of control and mastery
    d. Risk communication optimally is planned before a disaster occurs and includes communication during and after the event
    e. All of the above

CME Activity Evaluation—Enduring Material
Medical Society of the State of New York

Activity (Program) Name: *Hidden Impact: What You Need to Know for the Next Disaster: A Practical Mental Health Guide for Clinicians.*

Name of Authors: Committee on Disaster and Terrorism, Group for the Advancement of Psychiatry (GAP)

1. The stated objectives of this book were:

   ☐ Exceeded   ☐ Met   ☐ Not met

2. Will the knowledge learned in this book affect your practice?

   ☐ Very Much   ☐ Moderately   ☐ Minimally   ☐ None

3. Based on your participation in the CME activity, have you learned something that will change the way you practice medicine?

   ☐ Yes   Describe_____

   _____

   ☐ No   Why not?_____

   _____

   ☐ NA   Was this the wrong audience for this activity? _____

   _____

4. Did this CME activity inform you about: (list the actual objectives from your application)

   ☐ Yes   ☐ No   I will be able to appreciate how to prepare for and participate effectively in a disaster response within the existing disaster response framework.

   ☐ Yes   ☐ No   I have knowledge of the major agencies and organizations involved in disaster response and public health emergencies.

   ☐ Yes   ☐ No   I understand the importance of an array of mental health screening and assessment tools useful in disaster settings.

☐ Yes ☐ No   I appreciate the spectrum of normal and abnormal behavioral and emotional responses to disasters.

☐ Yes ☐ No   I appreciate the needs of special populations in disaster, including children.

☐ Yes ☐ No   I understand the pharmacological and psychological options and limitations in the post-disaster management of behavioral and emotional concerns.

☐ Yes ☐ No   I appreciate the elements of psychological first aid and its application in the disaster setting.

☐ Yes ☐ No   I appreciate the role of collaboration and consultation in the management of disaster-related mental health issues.

☐ Yes ☐ No   I appreciate the legal and ethical dimensions of disaster work.

☐ Yes ☐ No   I appreciate the importance of self-care during and after disaster.

☐ Yes ☐ No   I will be aware of the processes of resiliency and recovery in communities and individuals.

Topics for future editions of this book:

1._____

2._____

Would you consider participating in other activities to enhance the knowledge you acquired from this book?

☐ Yes ☐ No   Live training

☐ Yes ☐ No   Interactive CD-ROM

☐ Yes ☐ No   Webinar

☐ Yes ☐ No   Other: _____

THANK YOU FOR ASSISTING US IN EVALUATING THIS ACTIVITY!